Body Contouring - Surgical Procedures and New Technologies

Edited by Alexandro Aguilera

Published in London, United Kingdom

Body Contouring - Surgical Procedures and New Technologies
http://dx.doi.org/10.5772/intechopen.102236
Edited by Alexandro Aguilera

Contributors
Armin Rudolph Geisse, Klaus Rudolph Oppliger, Thomas Rudolph Oppliger, André Salval, Valerio Badiali, Salvatore Giordano, Ali Juma, Jamil Hayek, Simon Davies, Marcos Leal Brioschi, Soane Couto Menezes Lemos, Carlos Dalmaso Neto, Franciele De Meneck, Patricia Rodrigues Resende, Eduardo Borba Neves, Sherif Wasief, Alexandro Aguilera

First published in London, United Kingdom, 2023 by IntechOpen
IntechOpen is the global imprint of INTECHOPEN LIMITED, registered in England and Wales, registration number: 11086078, 5 Princes Gate Court, London, SW7 2QJ, United Kingdom

British Library Cataloguing-in-Publication Data
A catalogue record for this book is available from the British Library

Additional hard and PDF copies can be obtained from orders@intechopen.com

Body Contouring - Surgical Procedures and New Technologies
Edited by Alexandro Aguilera
p. cm.
Print ISBN 978-1-83768-041-2
Online ISBN 978-1-83768-042-9
eBook (PDF) ISBN 978-1-83768-043-6

Meet the editor

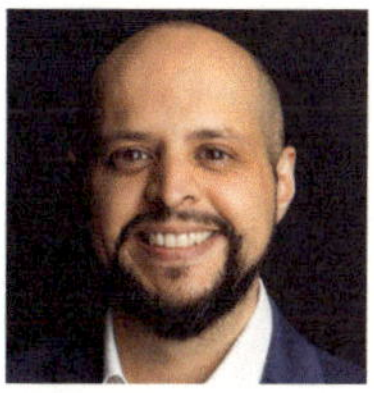

Dr. Alexandro Aguilera is a plastic and reconstructive surgeon and a faculty member of the Department of Plastic and Reconstructive Surgery, National Institute of Pediatrics, Mexico. He is board certified by the Mexican Board of Plastic, Aesthetic and Reconstructive Surgery. He completed a fellowship in hand surgery and another in facial palsy and peripheral nerves, both certified by the National Autonomous University of Mexico. Dr. Aguilera is a member of the Educational Committee of the Mexican Association of Plastic Surgeons and has contributed to several national and international plastic and reconstructive surgery meetings. He has numerous manuscripts, poster presentations, and books to his credit.

Contents

Preface **IX**

Section 1
Introduction **1**

Chapter 1 **3**
Introductory Chapter: New Horizons in Body Contouring
by Alexandro Aguilera

Section 2
Liposuction: State of the Art **7**

Chapter 2 **9**
Lipocontouring: Recipe for Esthetic Feminine Silhouette
by Sherif Wasief

Chapter 3 **23**
Body Contouring and VASER Technology, the Fourth Dimension
by Ali Juma, Jamil Hayek and Simon Davies

Section 3
Surgical Body Contouring **39**

Chapter 4 **41**
Perspective Chapter: Gluteal Augmentation with Complete Retromuscular Placement of Biconvex Silicone Implants
by Valerio Badiali, André Salval and Salvatore Giordano

Chapter 5 **53**
Perspective Chapter: Breast Reduction with Central Pedicle and Autologous Mesh Dermis – Surgical Tecnique
by Armin Rudolph Geisse, Klaus Rudolph Oppliger and Thomas Rudolph Oppliger

Section 4
Safety **69**

Chapter 6 **71**
Perspective Chapter: Identification of Body Contouring Surgery Complications by Multispectral RGB/Infrared Thermography Imaging
by Marcos Leal Brioschi, Soane Couto Menezes Lemos, Carlos Dalmaso Neto, Franciele De Meneck, Patricia Rodrigues Resende and Eduardo Borba Neves

Preface

Body contouring surgery has evolved greatly in the last decades. Along with cultural changes and new concepts of beauty, medical practice has also evolved following new ideas and patient expectations.

This book describes new techniques and devices, including surgical and nonsurgical procedures, in body contouring. It begins with a description of the evolution of liposuction. In the past, previous procedures were considered dangerous, resulting in poor outcomes and adverse side effects; patient safety was not a priority. As such, new technologies and care were needed, and a new term for liposuction emerged: liposculpture. There are various types of liposuction, ranging from soft or medium to high-definition liposuction, depending on how athletic a patient is and how much fat and skin laxity they have. The book also discusses preoperative markings for liposuction, which involves the surgeon marking the negative areas to work on to completely remove fat deposits, outlining the upper part of the midline, the lateral borders of the rectus abdominis muscle, the oblique and serratus muscles, and the iliac crest.

The second part of the book emphasizes some techniques for body contouring, starting with breast surgery. After the first breast implants became available, the initial trend was to use larger implants without considering the shape and readaptation of skin. Today, breast surgery has dramatically shifted, influenced by the type of activities modern patients engage in and with an eye towards shape and long-lasting results rather than just volume.

In patients who have had pregnancies or experienced weight fluctuations, a breast lift (mastopexy) may be needed, with or without the use of implants. The book describes some variations of the pedicles used in mastopexy in combination with the use of mesh in some instances or other options where the implants can be stabilized using a pre-pectoral pocket.

Next, the book discusses some new devices in body contouring. Power-assisted liposuction is an external device that generates an oscillatory movement in the canulae and hand piece that reduces the surgeon's fatigue, facilitating the extraction of more fat in less time. It is also a good tool for better defining the negative spaces in the abdomen. Other devices discussed include ultrasonic devices and internal radiofrequency devices that dilute fat and make its extraction easier, destroying adipose tissue and helping with the postoperative retraction of the skin. These devices achieve excellent definition of the worked areas with little inflammation and pain in the postoperative period, producing long-lasting results and allowing patients a more rapid return to their regular activities.

Finally, the book discusses skin resection, which is used if the patient has skin laxity and excess. Resection may range from a mini abdominoplasty to a complete or extended abdominoplasty or even a more advanced procedure called fleur-de-lis abdominoplasty, which is used in cases of skin excess and redundancy in the central and upper part of the abdomen. This procedure eliminates excess fat at the back, flanks, and lateral areas, helping to achieve a flat abdomen. The type of procedure used depends on the height and weight of the patient, the amount and extent of skin that needs to be resected, and the patient's general health. The book also discusses some safety specifications as they relate to these new technologies.

There is a promising future in body contouring procedures and it is important for surgeons to be aware of advancements in the field in order to keep up with and meet the needs and desires of patients.

Alexandro Aguilera
National Institute of Pediatrics,
Department of Peripheral Nerve and Hand Surgery,
Mexico City, Mexico

Section 1

Introduction

Chapter 1

Introductory Chapter: New Horizons in Body Contouring

Alexandro Aguilera

1. Introduction

The history of humanity and its scientific evolution cannot be described without pointing out the innate desire of our species to observe our surroundings, accompanied by the need to achieve better and consistent results through the invention of new technologies and devices. In the present days, these advances have come along also with the evolution of how patients see themselves, being more demanding than before, looking for less inflammation, shorter recovery periods, and natural and long-lasting results, following a modern vision of beauty mostly influenced by social media and ethnic parameters.

Regarding body contouring surgery, we have witnessed a massive change in the last few years, not only because of the cultural change in how patients see themselves and what types of bodies they are looking for, but also because of the new techniques and devices that have helped achieve those type of results modern patients want, and also because of a change of our own mentality we as surgeons have [1].

2. Cultural influence and patient expectations

First of all, the cultural changes have been very important to get us where we are standing nowadays. In the past, the type of results the patients often wanted was massively influenced by TV shows, movies, and magazines. With the boom of silicone breast implants, patients wanted to go as high in volume as they could, without considering the final shape and how they fit their general body contour as a whole, nor the effect of the weight will have in the breast, with the natural descent that comes in the following years. Nowadays, our patients have become more aware of their own bodies, looking for more natural and athletic looking results that can relate to the type of body of each patient, shifting our main vision in breast surgery influenced also with the type of activities modern female patients do, and looking for better shape and long-lasting results rather than just volume [2].

The same happened with their expectations from other body contouring procedures such as abdominoplasty and liposuction. From my point of view, this is one of the areas in plastic surgery with the most evolution in recent years. The general idea of the patients was just to take out volume from some areas, without volumizing others, or in other instances just remove the skin excess generated by pregnancies or by important changes in weight [3].

3. New technologies

Secondly, there has been a very important development in new technologies and devices. Practically each year we see a new console, a new machine that comes out to the market promising the best results. We as surgeons have to be very well informed on what effects those new technologies will produce in our patients, selecting which ones are best for them with consistent results and scientific evidence supporting them [4]. First, with the introduction of power-assisted liposuction, we as surgeons got less fatigued, with less movements we could extract a lot more of fat from a particular area, thus enhancing the results. Secondly came the ultrasonic liposculpture, helping us liquify the fat, eliminating the adipose tissue, facilitating the extraction, and helping us with the postoperative recovery with less inflammation and quicker recovery times. Finally, what we are using nowadays is operative radiofrequency helping us with a much better skin retraction, less inflammation, stimulation of collagen and elastin production, and with so, better skin quality and better results, enhancing negative areas and accentuating lights and shadows that make our results even better. The last piece in the puzzle has been the postoperative therapy that has helped the patient in a reduced swelling, less seromas formation, and better skin redraping to the areas where fat was extracted [5].

4. Surgeon's mindset

Finally, our mentality as plastic surgeons has also experienced an important change, focusing our practice in patient safety first, and with the support of the new technologies and advances previously described, the type of results we are looking for. In the past, previous procedures were even considered dangerous,

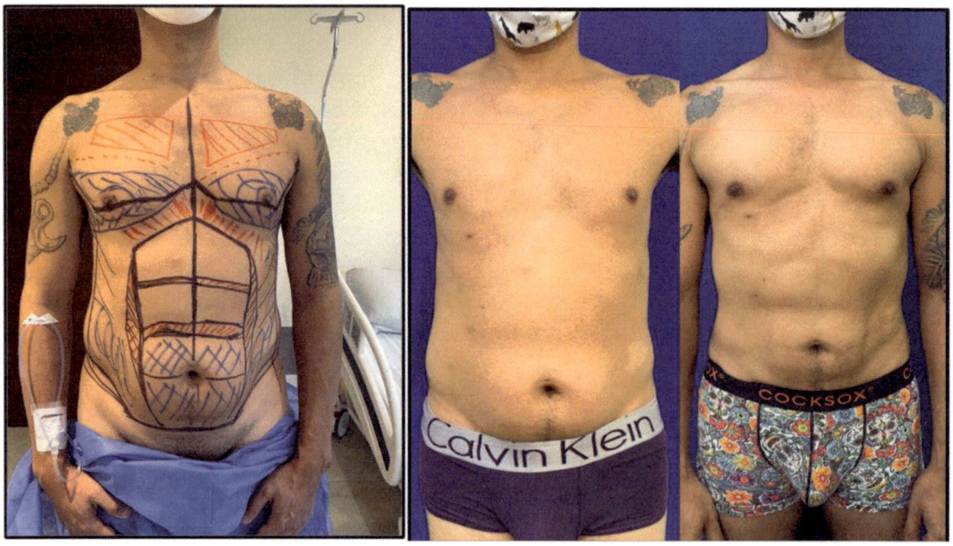

Figure 1.
A): Preoperative markings (in black we outline midlinemidline and lateral borders of rectus abdominis muscle in blue we outline the negative spaces to totally get rid of the fat in those compartments, and in red we outline the areas of fat transfer to enhance the pectoralis). B): Preoperative frontal picture. C): Postoperative picture after 6 months.

where patient safety was not a priority, resulting in dangerous side effects and very poor results. The second part of our mentality change is influenced also by cultural changes and the current definition of beauty, combined with a much better understanding of the male and female anatomy which in combination with the current technologies have helped us in achieving not only more natural results, but in selected patients high-definition results where we can enhance abdominal and back muscles, and even get athletic arms and legs, pectoral definition in men, treatment of gynecomastia, and in general a better body contour fit with the types of bodies we want (**Figure 1**).

In conclusion, there is a three-way responsibility in achieving better results, patients, new technologies, and surgeons. We need to have a better understanding of our patients' desires but also educate them on what can be done and what cannot, keep preparing ourselves in learning how to apply these technologies having in mind our patient's safety and how we can help them achieve the results they are looking for, helping them as we can with a better recovery period, less painful procedures, and quick return to their normal activities.

Author details

Alexandro Aguilera
National Institute of Pediatrics, Department of Peripheral Nerve and Hand Surgery, Mexico City, Mexico

*Address all correspondence to: alexandruss@hotmail.com

References

[1] Collins PS, Moyer KE. Evidence-based practice in liposuction. Annals of Plastic Surgery. 2018;**0**(00):1-3

[2] Chia CT, Neinstein, Theodorou. Evidence-based medicine: Liposuction. Plastic Reconstruction Surgery. 2017;**139**(1):267e-274e

[3] Mazzoni D, Lin J, Dubin, Khorasani. Review of non-invasive body contouring devices for fat reduction, skin tightening and muscle definition. The Australasian Journal of Dermatology. 2019;**60**(4):278-283

[4] Cárdenas-Camarena L, Reyes-Herrera, et al. Lipoabdominoplasty: What we have implemented and what we have modified over 26 years. Plastic and Reconstructive Surgery - Global Open. 2023;**11**:e4805. Pages: 1-13 [Published online 20 February 2023]

[5] Winocour J, Gupta V, Roberto Ramirez J, et al. Risk factors, complication rates, and safety of combined procedures. Plastic and Reconstructive Surgery. 2015;**136**:597e-606e

Section 2

Liposuction: State of the Art

Chapter 2

Lipocontouring: Recipe for Esthetic Feminine Silhouette

Sherif Wasief

Abstract

This chapter discusses the different types of procedures for augmenting body shape and size, including liposuction, lipoinjection, lipocontouring, and others. It presents a history and literature review of liposuction and details the author's personal techniques with accompanying figures and photographs. The chapter also discusses safety and common complications of body contouring techniques.

Keywords: lipocontouring, liposculpture, lipoinjection, hip-to-waist ratio, Brazilian butt lift (BBL), VASER, laser-assisted liposuction, expansion vibration lipoinjection (EVL), cellulite, buttock augmentation, thread lift

1. Introduction

The influence of social media on how people view their bodies is undeniable. Increasingly, many people consider an hourglass body shape with a narrow waist and round buttocks to be "ideal." This is true across many cultures and ethnic groups. Nowadays, there is a focus on buttock aesthetics, with many people wanting full, round buttocks free from cellulite and a small hip-to-waist ratio (**Figure 1**).

1.1 Liposuction, lipocontouring, and new concepts

Liposuction is one of the most frequently performed procedures in plastic surgery, accounting for 15–20% of all cosmetic procedures. In the last 5 years, it has been among the top three most requested procedures [1].

Contributions from researchers like Sterodimas, Coleman, Klein, Gasparotti, Zocchi, Apfelberg and others are the cornerstone for all current lipocontouring procedures performed [2–7].

Alfredo Hoyos and Peter Prendergast's book on high-definition liposculpture details advanced techniques in lipoplasty and autologous fat grafting [8]. The authors describe augmentation of muscular curves by lipoinjection over muscles and intramuscularly for an athletic body shape.

A meta-analysis by Hector Lázaro Cárdenas-Camarena et al [1] focused on safety and reducing fatal complications in liposuction. This study found that thromboembolic disease, fat embolism, pulmonary edema, lidocaine intoxication, and intraabdominal visceral lesion are the most serious complications when performing liposuction.

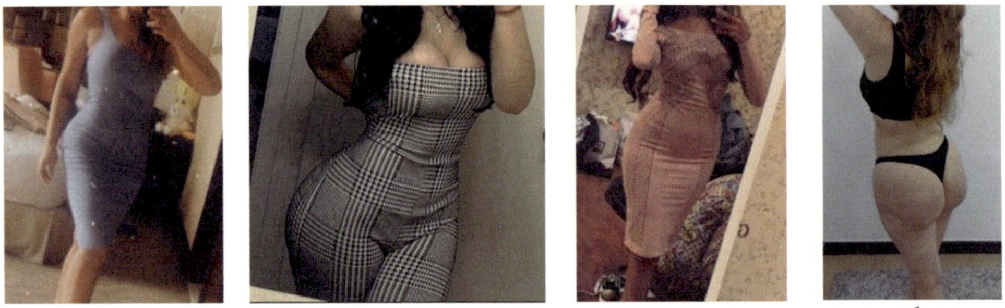

a b c d

Figure 1.
a, b, c and d are images of patients who have undergone lipocontouring; from different ethnicity.

Danilla described the rectus abdominis fat transfer (RAFT) technique, which involves transfer of fat directly to the rectus abdominis muscle after flap elevation during lipoabdominoplasty [9]. Gonzalez et al. investigated incorporating the ultrasound-guided rectus abdominis fat transfer (UGRAFT) technique after high-definition liposuction in one patient [10].

1.2 Gluteal fat augmentation

Strong et al. contributed to the refinement of the fat grafting procedure with their review of harvesting, processing, and injection techniques [11].

Luiz Toledo invented the "Brazilian Buttock Technique" for transferring fat to the buttocks [12].

Mendieta [13] published his classification of the liposculpture of the gluteal units for better understanding of the area; gluteal fat augmentation became a three-dimensional body contouring technique more than just a simple buttock augmentation; Mendieta described a gluteal esthetic unit classification system involving 10 units (see **Table 1** and **Figure 2**).

In Mendieta's classification system, six esthetic zones contribute to the buttock frame/shape: zones 1–5 and 8. The mid-lateral buttock (zone 8) is unique in that it

1.	**Sacrum v-zone**
2.	Flank
3.	Upper buttock
4.	Lower back
5.	Outer leg
6.	Gluteus
7.	Diamond zone: inner gluteal
8.	Mid-lateral buttock (point C)
9.	Inferior gluteal/posterior leg junction
10.	Upper back

Table 1.
Gluteal esthetic units.

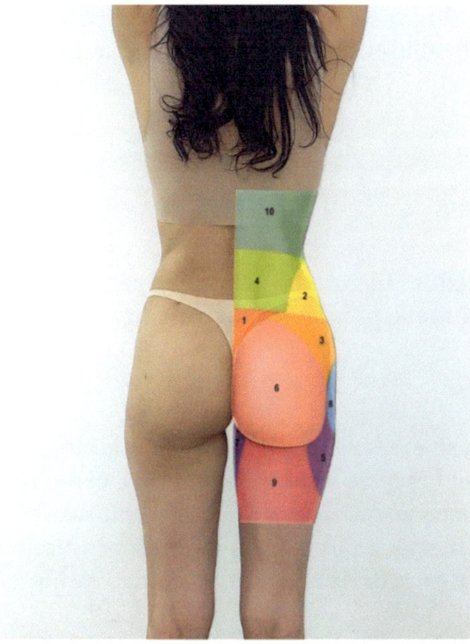

Figure 2.
Gluteal esthetic units.

often requires fat transfer to improve contour. Additionally, this area does not contain muscle and thus requires special attention and precision when fat grafting. All approaches involve liposuction of zones 1–4 in all patients. It is important to note that excessive liposuction of zone 5 can also lead to an unnatural transition zone between the buttock proper and the lateral thigh [14].

Expansion vibration lipofilling (EVL), first described by Del Vecchio and Wall, is a more efficient alternative to syringe-based injection in large-volume fat transplantation to the breast and buttock, employing basket cannulae and vibration through recipient site tissue. By utilizing 4-mm large-bore tubing, the authors demonstrated that large-volume fat transplantation procedures such as Brazilian butt lift (BBL) can be performed more expeditiously, free the operating hand from fatigue, and allow for more focus on cannula tip location and anatomic cannula depth [15].

2. Aim of this work

This case series demonstrates the effect of lipocontouring in female patients. We describe liposuction combined with lipoinjection to promote better understanding of the implementation of new technologies to maximize esthetic results while prioritizing safety.

A combination of liposuction of the back, waist, and abdomen with lipo-augmentation and liposculpture of the buttocks with treatment of cellulite and buttock lifting by threads produced good esthetic results and high rates of patient satisfaction.

3. Patients

This case series includes a cohort of 243 female patients aged 18–50 years with a body mass index (BMI) in the range of 18–40 who underwent lipocontouring and waist liposuction (lipo 360 procedure) combined with other surgeries such as buttock lipofilling, tummy tuck, cellulite treatment, and thread lifting of the buttocks.

4. Surgical technique

4.1 Medical history

Patients were screened for history of previous operations, diabetes mellitus, hypertension, use of blood thinners, pregnancies, smoking, and cardiovascular diseases.

4.2 Examination

Body shape, buttock shape, fat distribution, skin laxity, adhesion lines, intra-abdominal fat, abdominal muscle weakness, hernias, cellulite condition, stretch marks, scars and umbilicus were all examined. Patient waists were measured at the smallest (maximal indentation) point and patient hips were measured at the widest part. The measurements were divided to obtain waist-to-hip ratio.

4.3 Photography

Patients were photographed from shoulders to knees at a distance of 2 meters and from different angles: anteriorly at 45 degrees to the right and left, laterally on both sides, and posteriorly at 45 degrees to the right and left. Cellulite condition of the buttock area was photographed in both a state of relaxation and during muscle clenching.

4.4 Marking

Permanent markers were used to mark areas for deep and superficial liposuction, adhesion lines, areas for lipoinjection, and areas of cellulite.

And dynamic muscle lines definition.

4.5 Anesthesia

Both general and epidural anesthesia were used.

4.6 Patient positioning

Patients were placed prone then supine.

4.7 Liposuction: Video 1, https://bit.ly/3QHTY6c

4.7.1 Tumescent infiltration

Tranexamic acid (50 mg for 500 cc of Ringer's solution with maximum dose of 200 mg).

4.7.2 Suction-assisted liposuction (SAL)/traditional liposuction

No. 5 Mercedes cannula and no. 4 Basket cannula used for deep liposuction.
No. 4 Mercedes cannula used for superficial liposuction and dynamic lines.

4.7.3 Power-assisted liposuction (PAL)

No. 4 and no. 5 Mercedes cannulae.

4.7.4 Ultrasound-assisted liposuction (UAL)/VASER liposuction

VASER and LipoSound devices.
Used before liposuction.

4.7.5 Laser-assisted liposuction (LAL)

Fotona's Nd: YAG laser machine.
Used before liposuction.
In a few cases, we used the laser both before and after liposuction (sandwich technique).

4.7.6 Syringe liposuction

Toomey tip syringes mounted on toomey tip ready no. 4 Mercedes cannulae.

4.8 Fat processing and preparation

Fat was aspirated into sterile 2000-cc containers or into toomey tipped syringes.
Decantation was performed only if fat was yellow in color.
Wash of aspirated fat with Ringer's solution if bloody.

4.9 Lipoinjection: Video 1, https://bit.ly/3QHTY6c

No intramuscular injections were used in this series. Instead, only deep and superficial subcutaneous lipoinjections were used accordingly.

4.9.1 Syringe lipoinjection

Tommy tip syringes mounted on no. 4 Mercedes cannulae.
Three Luer lock syringes on no. 3 and no. 2 single-hole cannulae.

4.9.2 Expansion vibration Lipoinjection (EVL)

There is no propeller machine available in our practice and thus we used Toomey tipped syringes connected to a sterile single-use tube attached to a no. 4 Mercedes cannula.

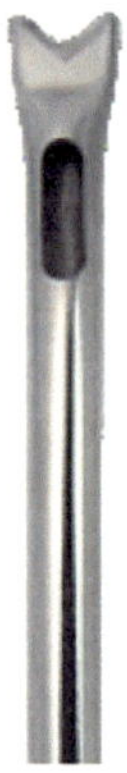

Figure 3.
V-tip/Toledo cannula.

Lipo-injection using power machine while vibration is on, another step of redistribution of fat after completion of lipoinjection by moving the cannula confirming homogenous redistribution of fat.

4.9.3 Cellulite release and C-point release: Video 2, https://bit.ly/3QHTY6c

Before lipoinjection the cellulite bands and adherent C-zone are prepared by injecting tumescent solution and cellulite bands and adhesions in c-point are released by no. 2 and/or no. 4 V-tip Toledo Cannula (**Figure 3**).

4.9.4 Ultrasound guidance during lipoinjection

Multiple safety reports and task forces have banned gluteal intramuscular lipoinjection. Several papers reported accidental intramuscular injections despite the surgeon's intentions to inject subcutaneously. Using ultrasound during injection increases precision and safety (**Figure 4**).

4.9.5 Thread lifting

Figure 5 shows the author's personal thread lifting procedure using a no. 1 polydioxanone (PDS) loop suture, which is used in patients with skin laxity who refuse surgical lifting as purse string suture with 2 passages.

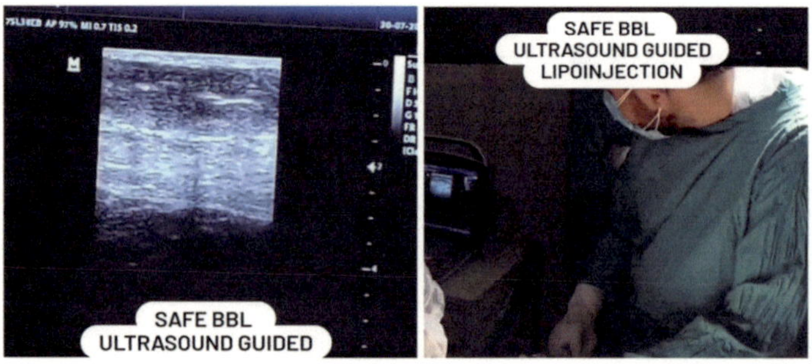

Figure 4.
Ultrasound-assisted lipoinjection of buttocks.

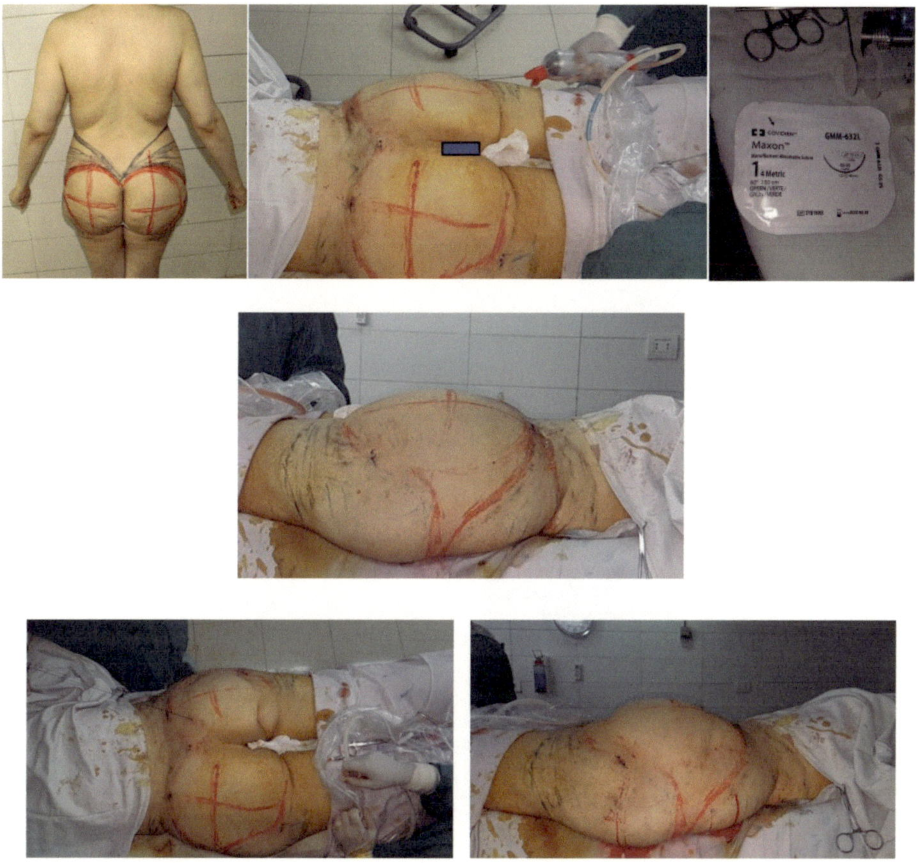

Figure 5.
Thread lifting of buttocks (author's personal technique).

5. Results

5.1 Patient presentation: Video 3, https://bit.ly/3QHTY6c

Figure 6 shows the results of VASER liposuction (1000 cc) and syringe lipoinjection (700 cc of purified fat re-injected) in a 40-year-old patient weighing 55 kilograms.

5.2 Patient presentation

Figure 7 shows the results of VASER liposuction (4000 cc) and EVL lipofilling (2000 cc of purified fat re-injected) in a 40-year-old patient weighing 72 kilograms.

5.3 Patient presentation

Figure 8 shows the results of tummy tuck, traditional liposuction (5000 cc), and syringe lipoinjection (1000 cc of purified fat re-injected) in a 42-year-old patient weighing 75 kilograms.

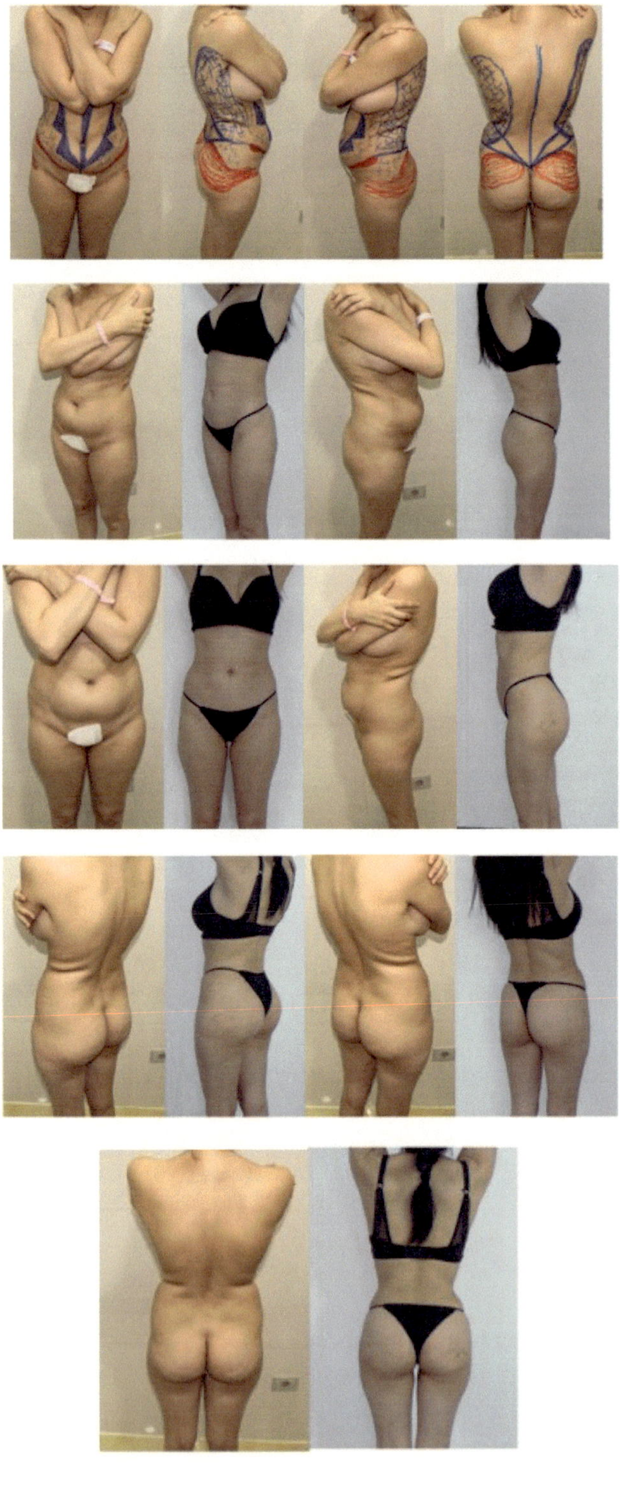

Figure 6.
Preoperative marking and postoperative photos of lipocontouring in a 40-year-old patient weighing 55 kilograms.

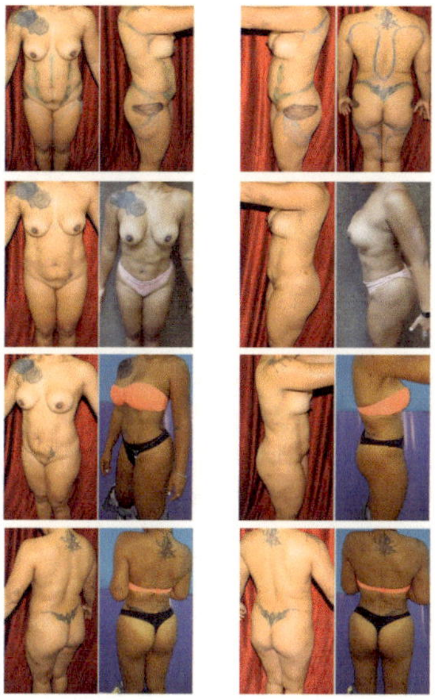

Figure 7.
Preoperative, marking and post operative photos of lipocontouring in 40 years 72 kilograms patient.

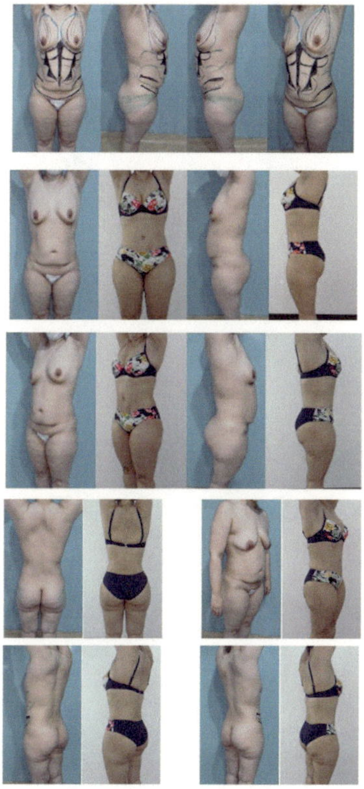

Figure 8.
Preoperative marking and postoperative photos of lipocontouring in a 42-year-old patient weighing 75 kilograms.

6. Discussion

Technology and medical knowledge in all fields of plastic surgery, especially body contouring, have expanded tremendously in the last years. The number of patients, plastic surgeons, and procedures is increasing with market expansion.

This chapter discussed our contouring technique, which is easy to learn, simple, and reproducible. In addition, it has a high satisfaction rate and low complication rate.

Adding energy devices to the armamentarium of plastic surgeons, and using them with caution and within safety limits after sufficient training, leads to improved results with smoother curves and better skin re-draping.

Skin burns and vascular insults of the skin are the major complications reported in the literature. These may occur in small areas (e.g., loins) where straight cannulae hit directly into the skin. One patient in our series had bilateral burns after treatment with the LipoSound device (**Figure 9**).

Larger burns and necrosis of larger areas of skin have also been reported in the literature [16]. No major burns occurred in this series.

Skin scarring and discoloration have also been reported, the latter being a more common occurrence. These complications can be largely avoided via cautious use of energy devices during liposuction (**Figure 10**).

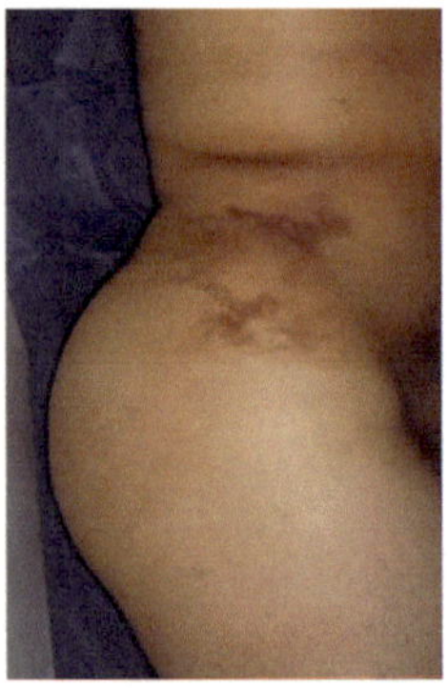

Figure 9.
Bilateral burns in a patient after undergoing treatment with LipoSound device.

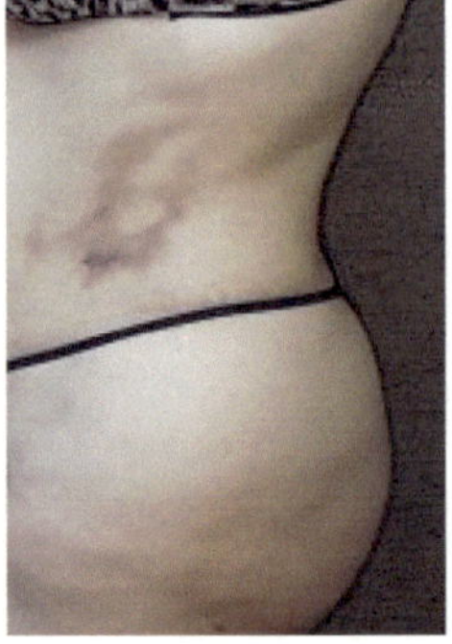

Figure 10.
Pigmented scarring in a patient after undergoing treatment with LipoSound device.

Blood transfusions may be necessary when using liposuction to remove large amounts of fat or when there is excessive bleeding. Other complications may include skin irregularities and over and under corrections.

Teamwork among anesthesiologists, nursing staff, assisting surgeons, and residents is essential for safety and efficacy of body contouring procedures.

7. Conclusion

Lipocontouring procedures can help patients obtain their desired body shape and size. For some patients, this may mean a narrower waist, smaller waist-to-hip ratio, smooth transition from waist to hip, better skin tone, or less cellulite in the buttock area. The procedures used are based on patient factors such as bony frame, skin quality, age, health status, smoking condition, and amount of weight and fat resources. Differences in these factors among patients give different results. Although the best result is usually obtained with the initial surgery, some patients may opt for secondary and revisionary surgeries. For example, an additional round of fat grafting to the buttocks may produce a more esthetic result.

Acknowledgements

I am grateful for the opportunity to discuss ideas, ask questions, and receive input and guidance from Dr. Luiz Toledo, Dr. Hector Duran, and Dr. Carlos Oaxaca.

Ultrasound lipoinjections were guided by my anesthesia consultant Dr. Ahmed Shehab.

Conflict of interest

"I declare no conflict of interest."

Notes/thanks/other declarations

I would like to thank my mom, dad, wife, and children for their support and sacrifice as I worked to complete this chapter. Special thanks to my team, especially my resident Dr. Hadeer el Shazly for her invaluable assistance.

Author details

Sherif Wasief
Shark El Madina Hospital, Alexandria, Egypt

*Address all correspondence to: sherif_wasief@yahoo.com

References

[1] Cárdenas-Camarena L, Andrés Gerardo LP, Durán H, Bayter-Marin JE. Strategies for reducing fatal complications in liposuction. Plastic and Reconstructive Surgery. Global Open. 2017;**5**(10):e1539

[2] Sterodimas A, Boriani F, Magarakis E, Nicaretta B, Pereira LH, Illouz YG. Thirtyfour years of liposuction: Past, present and future. European Review for Medical and Pharmacological Sciences. 2012;**16**(3):393-406

[3] Coleman WP 3rd. The history of liposuction and fat transplantation in America. Dermatologic Clinics. 1999;**17**(4):723-727

[4] Klein JA. The tumescent technique. Anesthesia and modified liposuction technique. Dermatologic Clinics. 1990;**8**(3):425-437

[5] Gasparotti M, Lewis CM, Toledo LS. Superficial liposuction: A new application of the technique for aged and flaccid skin. Aesthetic Plastic Surgery. Spring 1992;**16**(2):141-153. DOI: 10.1007/BF00450606. PMID: 1570777

[6] Zocchi M. Ultrasonic liposculpturing. Aesthetic Plastic Surgery. 1992;**16**(4):287-298

[7] Apfelberg DB. Results of multicenter study of laser-assisted liposuction. Clinics in Plastic Surgery. 1996;**23**(4):713-719

[8] Hoyos A, Prendergast PM. High Definition Body Sculpting. Berlin An: Springer-Verlag; 2016

[9] Danilla S. Rectus abdominis fat transfer (RAFT) in lipoabdominoplasty: A new technique to achieve fitness body contour in patients that require tummy tuck. Aesthetic Plastic Surgery. 2017;**41**(6):1389-1399

[10] Flores González EA, Viaro MSS, Duran Vega HC, Ramírez Guerrero OR, Brito Toledo P, Vázquez Apodaca RA, et al. Incorporation of the UGRAFT technique to high-definition liposuction. Plastic and Reconstructive Surgery. Global Open. 2022;**10**(7):e4447. DOI: 10.1097/GOX.0000000000004447

[11] Strong AL, Cederna PS, Rubin JP, Coleman SR, Levi B. The current state of fat grafting: A review of harvesting, processing, and injection techniques. Plastic and Reconstructive Surgery. 2015;**136**(4):897-912

[12] Toledo LS. Gluteal augmentation with fat grafting: The Brazilian buttock technique: 30 years' experience. Clinics in Plastic Surgery. 2015;**42**(2):253-261

[13] Mendieta CG. Gluteal reshaping. Aesthetic Surgery Journal. 2007;**27**(6):641-655

[14] Del Vecchio DA, Wall SJ Jr, Mendieta CG, Aslani AA, Hoyos AE, Mallucci PL, et al. Safety comparison of Abdominoplasty and Brazilian butt lift: What the literature tells us. Plastic and Reconstructive Surgery. 2021;**148**(6):1270-1277

[15] Hoyos AE, Duran H, Cardenas-Camarena L, Bayter JE, Cala L, Perez M, et al. Use of Tranexamic acid in Liposculpture: A double-blind, multicenter. Randomized Clinical Trial. Plast Reconstr Surg. 2022;**150**(3):569-577

[16] Dixit VV, Wagh MS. Unfavourable outcomes of liposuction and their management. Indian J Plast Surg. 2013;**46**(2):377-392. DOI: 10.4103/0970-0358.118617

Chapter 3

Body Contouring and VASER Technology, the Fourth Dimension

Ali Juma, Jamil Hayek and Simon Davies

Abstract

Body contouring surgery encompasses several facets. However, it is only in the last 15 years that body-sculpting technology has been incorporated in body contouring on a larger scale. This has added further refinements to the aesthetic outcomes of body contouring surgery. Advances in VASER technology meant it has become synonymous with the art of lipo-sculpture, body sculpting and body contouring. When performing body contouring, the first step in liposculpturing the tissues is to emulsify the fat using ultrasound resonance. The emulsified fat is then aspirated with a power-assisted suction device, and in appropriately selected patients, surgically excising the skin excess to achieve the desired results. It is important not to forget the other added bonuses of VASER technology, which includes reduced surgeon's fatigue, enhanced skin retraction and reduced downtime; all being achieved at a high safety margin. Body contouring does not stop at emulsifying fat and aspirating it. Fat transfer in the selected patients has become an integral part of body contouring surgery. This includes patients wishing breast augmentation and buttock augmentation utilising their own fat, thereby reducing any concerns they may have with using silicone-based implants, whilst achieving cosmetically pleasing long-lasting outcomes. Surgical excision where technology cannot overcome skin excess and laxity adds to the aesthetic outcomes in selected cases, thus bringing to fruition the hybrid surgical approach popularised in the twenty-first century. One example of many is incorporating VASER lipo-sculpture with abdominoplasty.

Keywords: body contouring, VASER, lipo-sculpture, abdominoplasty, body sculpting, fat transfer, aesthetic outcomes

1. Introduction

Contouring is defined as the action of changing the shape of something [1] (Cambridge English Dictionary). However, in a Plastic Surgeon's eyes, it is the action of forming and shaping new cosmetically pleasing contours of the body or face. In doing so, thus recreating and restoring the desirable anatomical relationships nearest to the golden ratio of beauty yet respecting the racial differences of beauty.

One of the great doyens of Plastic surgery, Ivo Pitanguy defined body contouring surgery as a collection of procedures with the goal of volumetric manipulation of superficial tissue, normally the adipose tissue, with or without removal of skin excess [2].

In our opinion, body contouring is the foundation of recreating beauty by moulding tissues, proportioning contours and removing excess, be it fat and/or skin when applicable. This recreates positive 'spaces' (light reflection) and negative spaces (shadows) when warranted and where desired (**Figure 1**). We must always remember that the patient's realistic goals and aspirations must be an integral part of our plans in achieving the best results.

Although technologies have added to the outcomes in body contouring, it is of profound importance to remember that it is unlikely to replace surgery in entirety and certainly not for the near foreseeable future. However, it will remain a powerful adjunct to surgery raising the bar to achieve consistent good outcomes in body contouring especially when using the hybrid approach.

The expectations of the human body-form appearance in both sexes have changed over the last five decades. This evolution is in continuous flux and in our opinion, is heavily influenced by factors including social media and designs of attire. This adds significant peer pressures to both patient and plastic surgeon alike.

Peer pressure on the surgeon has its drawbacks, but also has its benefits. One such important benefit is driving advances in our speciality in safe surgical techniques and technologies. This spurs on the medical technology companies influenced by market forces to continually respond to the demands of the plastic surgeon based in part on patient's aspirations.

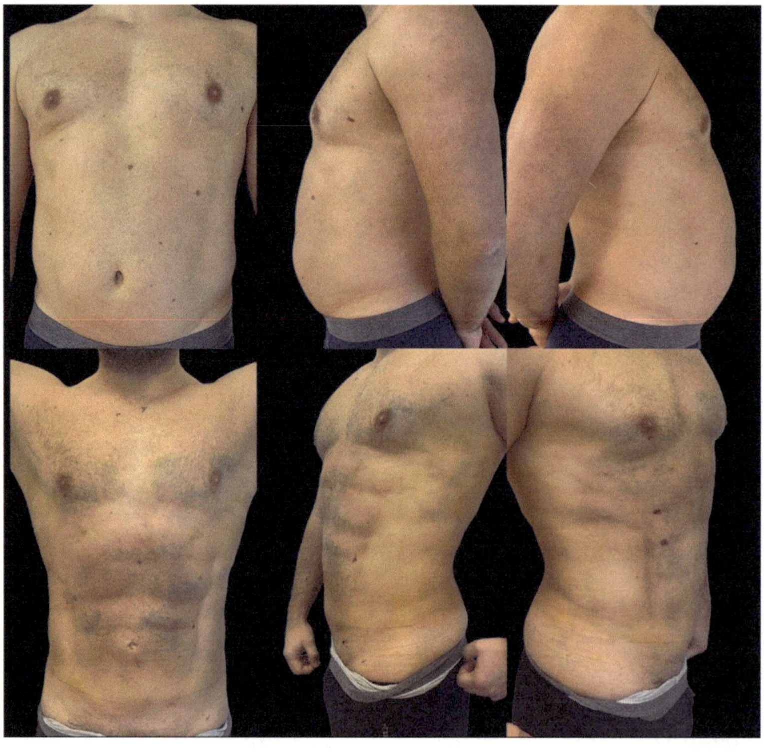

Figure 1.
Forty-two-year-old male who had undergone high-definition body sculpting with VASER. The lipoaspirate was 4.4 litres.

2. Technologies in body contouring

The technology in body contouring continues to evolve. The devices on the market are numerous; however, as the chapter is designated to talk about VASER technology, body contouring and the hybrid approach, hence, we will concentrate our writing on this technology, its role and relationship with surgery in body contouring.

What does VASER stand for? It is an acronym, which stands for 'Vibration Amplification of Sound Energy at Resonance'. Certainly, a scientific mouthful, which practically can be simplified through describing its action in plain English. The ultrasound waves break up and liquefy fat cells making it easier to remove by liposuction at lower pressures with ease and more abundance than with traditional methods. In doing so reducing surgeon's fatigue yet safely achieving consistent aesthetic outcomes, thus popularising this type of body contouring surgery (**Figure 1**).

3. The evolution of VASER

Ultrasound-assisted liposuction (UAL) broke down fat cells to produce an emulsion, leading to a less traumatic aspiration of fat. Unfortunately, early on high incidence of burns, skin necrosis and scarring occurred [3, 4].

The development of hollow probes rather than the earlier solid probes although meant less risks; however, the high energy delivered meant when used near to skin; burns, scarring, waviness and contour irregularities could occur [3, 4].

The first report of clinical application of a third-generation ultrasound liposculpture device, which used pulsed low-power ultrasound and high-efficiency small-diameter solid titanium probes; VASER liposculpture was reported by Jewell et al. [5]. The energy was much less and the pulsed mode reduced heat generation, thus reducing risks and potential complications.

The advent of VASER meant plastic surgeons elevated liposuction to new highs, and VASER-assisted liposculpture (VAL) became popularised. Alfredo Hoyos embraced this technology from an early stage and pushed the boundaries to new levels [6].

With these advances was born new nomenclature formulated to describe the complexity of the detailed sculpting of the superficial fat and deep fat over muscles and in between muscles VAHDL [7].

4. The evolution of fat transfer

Fat grafting and lipofilling are synonymous with fat transfer. In this chapter, we will use the term fat transfer, as in our opinion it is more fitting as a descriptive term than either of the other two; however, the words may be used interchangeably.

Fat transfer was first documented in 1889 when omental fat was grafted between the liver and diaphragm to repair a diaphragmatic hernia [8].

In 1892, Neuber et al. described fat taken from the forearm and transferred to fill a volume and contour irregularity of the face caused by a scar with excellent results [9].

In 1895, Czerny et al. transferred fat from a lipoma of the back for breast reconstruction [10].

The first needle and syringe fat transfer was demonstrated by Brunning et al. in 1911 when he injected for the first-time fat subcutaneously in the nose to correct the aesthetic result following rhinoplasty. Brunning was the first to identify that fat resorption meant the results were not sustainable [11].

Refinements of the fat transfer did not occur until 1975 when the Fischers, father and son, developed the modern techniques of liposuction using metal cannulas [12].

Further advancements in liposuction and fat transfer techniques occurred when in 1992 Coleman proposed a new method of harvesting fat, which minimised trauma to adipocytes [13].

In 1993, Klein added the Tumescent technique which made harvesting fat easier and less traumatic to the adipocytes with less blood loss making large volume fat harvesting possible with a higher safety margin; this popularised large volume liposuction [14].

In our opinion, with the advent of safer large volume fat harvesting, it was only natural that the collected fat ought not go to waste, hence paving the way to large volume fat transfer.

5. Fat donor and recipient sites, our experience

In this chapter, we will consider the donor sites we commonly harvest fat from and the recipient anatomical sites we transfer fat to. In our series the recipient of fat most common anatomical sites included the face, breasts, and buttocks. This parallels what is documented in the world literature [15].

Our choice of fat donors site/s depends on a number of factors including the amount of fat required, the anatomical area we plan to transfer the fat to, and the anatomical location/s where fat is available especially in the thin patient. We must respect that in harvesting the fat; the donor site/s aesthetic outcomes are appropriately proportioned.

Since we started liposculpturing the body's different anatomical sites with Vaser, it has become much easier to make available the amount of fat required to transfer to breasts and buttocks when other less advanced methods fail at worst or at best may not achieve this in one stage. In our experience, this is not so for the face as the volumes required are relatively small and, in most cases, available even with less advanced technology. In the face and in the majority, we tend to use syringe-assisted lipo-aspiration to harvest the fat for transfer.

6. Face contouring

When transferring fat to the face or anatomical areas of the face, we tend to use submental fat if available (**Figures 2–4**), including when performing a facelift. In the case when submental fat is of limited availability, then we use abdominal fat.

In the case of fat transfer to breasts and buttocks, we use the abdomen, lower back and thighs. The thighs are used as a backup unless the preoperative plan included them as a part of body contouring.

In the face and in selected patients, fat transfer can be used as a sole method of facial rejuvenation instead of dermal, Hyaluronic Acid, fillers (**Figure 5**). Fat can also be used an adjunct to face and midface lift surgery, thus adding further refinement to the cosmetic outcomes.

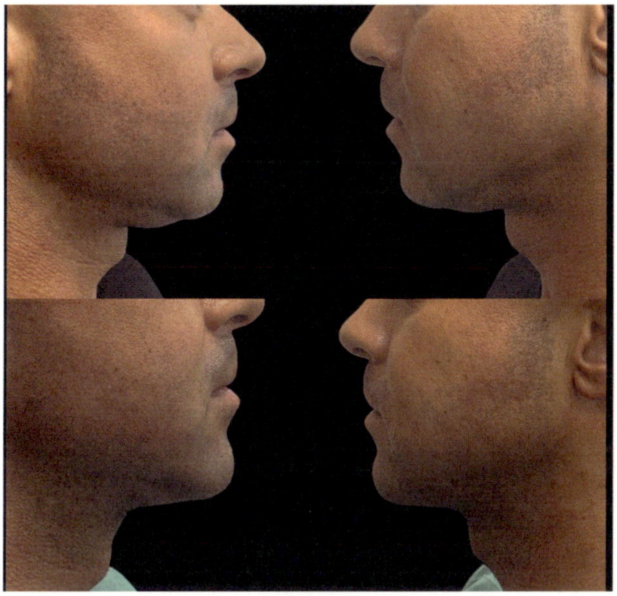

Figure 2.
Twenty-nine-year-old male 7 months following VASER liposuction of neck and 6 cc fat transfer of fat to chin.

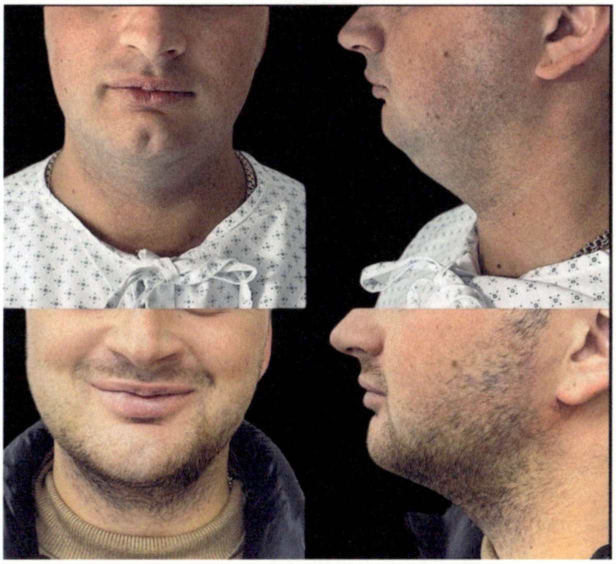

Figure 3.
Thirty-four-year-old male 3 weeks following submental and neck liposuction in addition to buccal fat removal. An 8 cc fat transfer to chin was also performed.

Fat is injected in key areas of the face including the temples, zygomatic area/ cheeks, midface, nasolabial folds, lateral cheeks, pre-jowl sulcus, marionette lines and jawline. The glabella, brows and forehead are also targeted sites for fat transfer in selected patients (**Figure 5**). Our plans when transferring fat into the face or any of its anatomical areas mirror, the techniques we use when injecting hyaluronic acid dermal fillers in the ageing face (**Figures 2–4**).

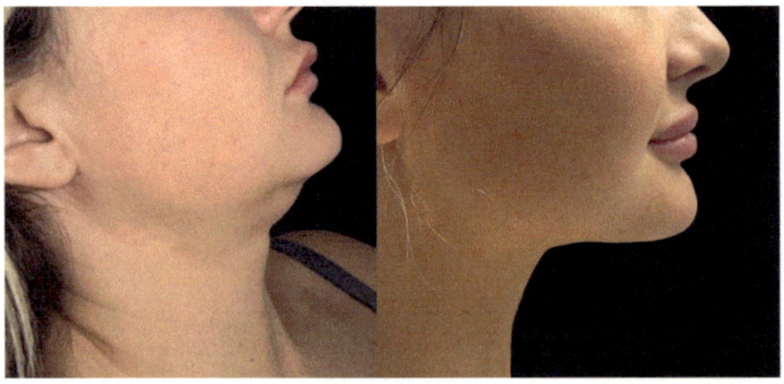

Figure 4.
Twenty-eight-year-old female 1 week following neck liposuction, buccal fat removal and 2 cc fat transfer to chin.

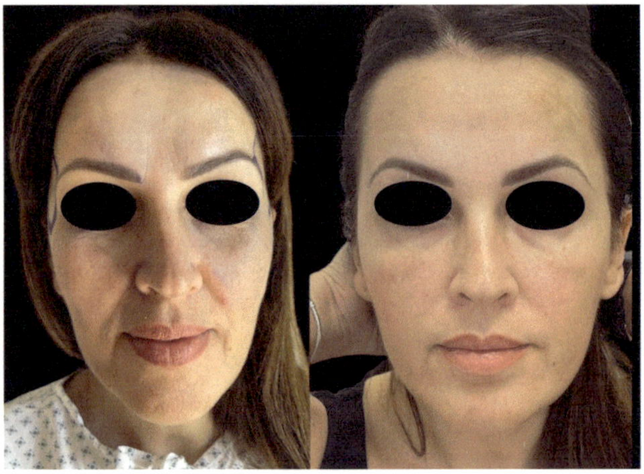

Figure 5.
Fifty-one-year-old female 5 months following 24 cc of fat transfer to face.

When transferring fat to the face, we methodically target the different planes injecting different consistency of fat in the different compartments, both the superficial and deep fat compartments [16], in addition to depositing the fat on the bone when required.

Our non-surgical dermal fillers experience in injecting the face contributed to us pushing the boundaries with our fat transfer techniques further adding to the aesthetic outcomes of our patients.

We developed a simple formula relating to the amount of fat required to be transferred in face rejuvenation. One millilitre (1 cc) of hyaluronic acid filler equates to 2-3 cc of fat irrespective of age or anatomical area.

However, we must keep in mind that fat does not have the same lifting properties as hyaluronic acid and different anatomical areas require different consistency of fat and viscosity. One such example is Nano-fat in the tear trough and lower eyelids area [17]. We use mechanical agitation to obtain this type of fat following its harvest.

In the twenty-first century, we feel that using high-definition ultrasound is likely to be the next step in progression when transferring fat into the face, thus aiding the accurate placement of fat, helping to avoid blood vessels, thus further reducing risks.

DOI: http://dx.doi.org/10.5772/intechopen.108935

7. Abdominal contouring

Our algorithm for abdominal contouring is simple. It pivots on four determining factors.

The first factor is the skin quality, laxity and excess. The second the rectus sheath its weakness, bulge, divarication and any hernia/s. The third is fat, its excess and distribution. The fourth is patients' aspirations and whether they are achievable, if so, how best to achieve them safely and efficiently.

If the skin quality is poor with laxity and significant excess, then a surgical excision is warranted (**Figure 6**). If the rectus sheath shows weakness with bulge and divarication, a plication is required. If a hernia is detected on ultrasound prior to surgery, then a multidisciplinary repair of this hernia with a general surgeon is planned.

Fat excess warrants liposculpture; however, the fat distribution influences the way we create curves and the time it takes. Patients' aspirations will have an influence on us as plastic surgeons; however, we must respect the confines of what is scientifically achievable within the realms of safety yet obtaining the best aesthetic results.

We must on occasions when a patient has unrealistic expectations protect that patient by being honest with them. Although we let them down gently, however, we will offer them the reasoning as to why and the support required.

Abdominoplasty with rectus sheath plication is a common procedure. Our aspirations and goals are to push the surgical outcomes of abdominoplasty to new heights. This is achievable when the aesthetic results of surgery; significantly outweighs the size of scarring whilst creating the desired contours and appropriate proportions. To do so, an open mind utilising a hybrid approach must be contemplated (**Figures 7** and **8**).

As plastic surgeons we aspire to always better our surgical outcomes and improve safety. Understanding the abdominal vascular territories and blood supply meant we could incorporate liposculpture with surgical excision yet reduce surgical complications [18].

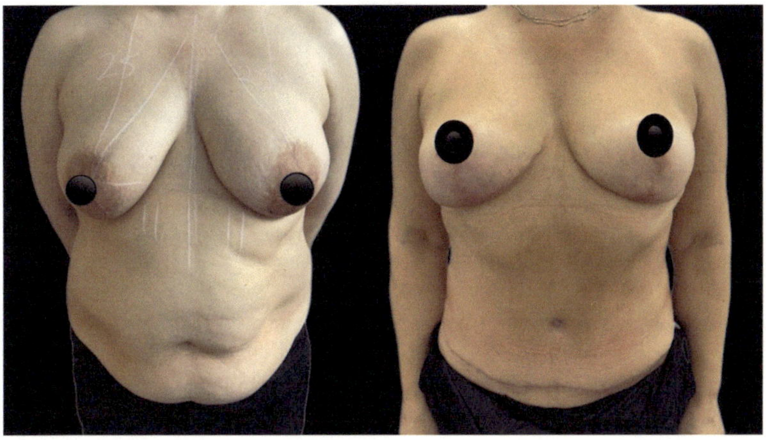

Figure 6.
Forty-nine-year-old female 6 months following VASER liposculpture to abdomen and flanks with abdominoplasty and plication of the rectus sheath. She also had bilateral breast reduction with fat transfer to upper poles to improve upper pole fullness.

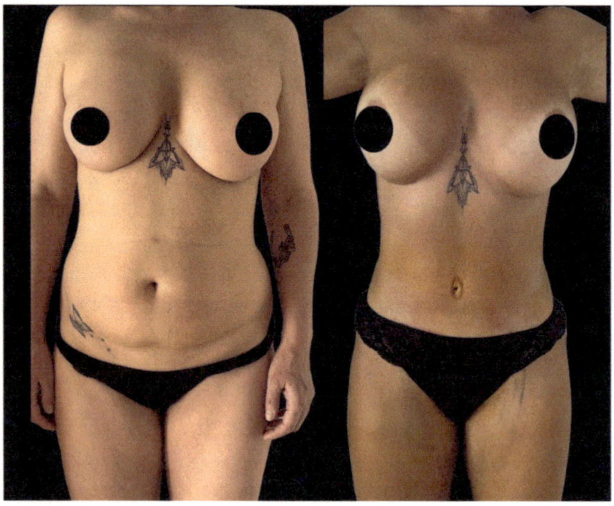

Figure 7.
Forty-three-year-old female 6 months following 360 VASER liposculpture of abdomen and flanks with first stage fat transfer to breasts. Followed by a second stage VASER liposculpture of thighs and back.

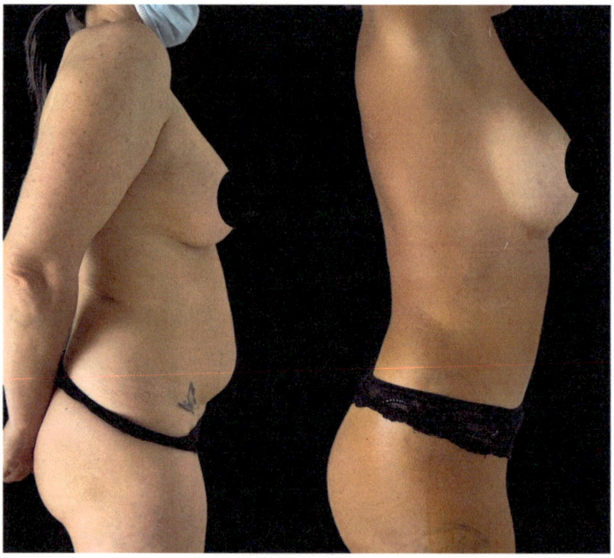

Figure 8.
Forty-three-year-old female 6 months following 360 VASER liposculpture of abdomen, and flanks with first stage fat transfer to breasts. Followed by a second stage VASER liposculpture of thighs and back.

VASER has added a safety margin to abdominoplasty as it produces less traumatic fat removal from the abdominal flap, thus decreasing the chances of complications associated with lipo-abdominoplasty [19].

Suction-assisted liposuction does not impair the regenerative potential of adipose-derived stem cells [20]. As the lipo-aspiration pressures are much lower following VASER than traditional liposuction, this also reduces risks to the skin [21].

The Vent-X, which is the vacuum pump designed to work with VASER, the vacuum it generates ranges from 0 to 760 mmHg. The dial starts at zero and goes all the way to 30. If we are to perform lipo-aspiration with fat transfer in mind, then we set the dial at 10–12, which equates to a third of atmosphere, ~250 mmHg. In doing so, we protect the skin and the harvested fat [21]. VASER also reduces surgeon's fatigue as the more fluid fat the easier it is to aspirate.

The time it takes from fat harvest to fat transfer has a bearing on the retention of fat in the recipient site. The shorter the time, the better the uptake with a critical period of 2 hours [22]. With VASER making fat harvest more time-efficient, this could further aid in better fat retention.

We must consider whether there is a limit of the lipoaspirate volume when performing an abdominoplasty; however, overall, the literature appears to support that current limits on liposuction volumes in lipo-abdominoplasty are arbitrary and do not reflect valid thresholds for increased complications in the hands of an experienced plastic surgeon [23].

8. Breast contouring

Accepting when we think of the word breast/s contouring does not normally stem to mind. When talking about breast contouring in the majority, we tend to focus on augmentation, reduction, mastopexy and mastopexy augmentation. However, if we go back to the basics, the word contouring is to change the shape of something, hence by changing the shape of the breast/s we are effectively contouring them [24–26].

Fat transfer to the breasts has become popularised following a change in the views about its safety by the American Society of Plastic Surgeons in 2009. It was more than two decades when they condemned this procedure due to fear that it may obscure the detection of breast cancer [24–26].

In this section, we will focus on breast contouring and fat transfer in the context of autogenous augmentation, mastopexy augmentation, asymmetry correction, and volume replacement (**Figure 9**).

The hybrid approach, which includes silicone implants with fat transfer, will also be considered. In selected patients, fat transfer is performed at the same time as breast reduction surgery; thus, adding fullness to the upper poles and cleavage of the breasts (**Figure 6**).

We must accept that not all patients desire one or the other treatment/s and fat is not always available to achieve the goals set out in the agreed pre-treatment planning schedule.

Considerations when injecting fat in the breasts include targeting the subcutaneous space and pre-pectoral plane, in addition to the breast tissue. Respecting the views of others and their practices, however, we do not see a case for transferring fat into or under the pectoral muscles and feel that this could add unnecessary risks without necessarily improving the aesthetic outcomes.

It is important to keep in mind that the pre-operative breasts' volume has an influence on the volume that ought to be transferred. Hence, it is important to appropriately counsel the patients prior to treating them as fat resorption will occur and can vary between 30 and 70% of the transferred volume within 12 months of transfer [27].

In females who are undergoing fat transfer to the breasts, we include a routine mammogram as a baseline in patients ≥40 years of age. As an added safety net, we routinely perform abdominal ultrasound screening if we are using the abdomen as a fat donor site to exclude any clinically undetected hernias and rectus sheath pathology or abnormal anatomy.

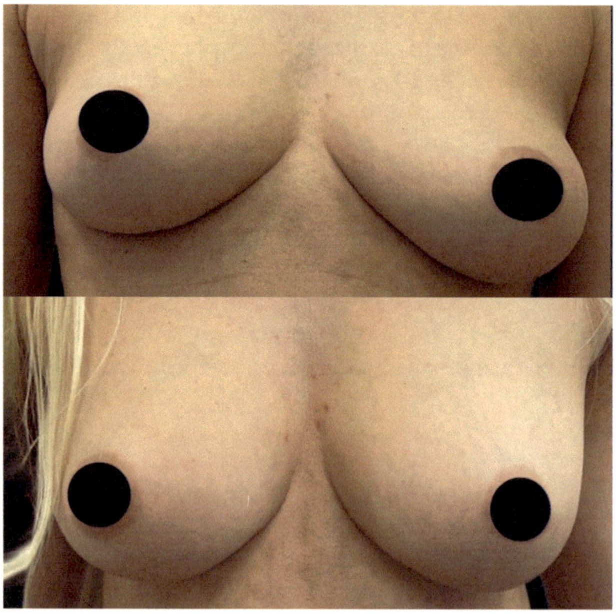

Figure 9.
Thirty-year-old female. She had VASER liposculpture to abdomen. She had 340 cc of fat transferred to right breast and 220 cc to left breast for the purpose of asymmetry correction and augmentation.

Surgical fat transfer techniques include three steps, fat harvest, processing the harvested fat and finally injecting it into the breast/s [28].

The volume of fat required influences the technique for fat harvesting. Early on we used a syringe-based mechanical aspiration of the fat and the Coleman centrifuge [29].

However, we now use Vaser for the larger volume fat harvest with a 3.7 mm cannula. Our technique includes allowing the aspirated fat to self-separate over a period of 30 minutes rather than spinning it with centrifuge, as we believe this reduces the trauma to the harvested fat.

The fat is then injected into the breasts using a 10 cc syringe and 2 mm cannula. For further refinement, a 5 or 1 cc syringe can be used when required.

Although the literature supports the view that when using the larger harvest cannula, the more fat survives. Nonetheless, a balance must be struck between cosmetic outcomes and scarring extent [30].

Our experience tells us like others that the less we handle the fat, the better is the survival rate when transferred into other tissues [31].

It is important to add that it is best to transfer the fat without significant time delay from the time it was harvested and to use a closed system when harvesting the fat with the least exposure to air [32].

The fat must be infused with small volume injections and distributed in different levels of the breast with the least traumatic method using a retrograde injection technique to minimise injections into vascular spaces. We aspire to limit the fat transfer volume per breast to 250–300 cc (**Figures 6** and 7).

If larger volume of fat is required for transfer in a small breast, then pre-surgery external expansion is recommended [33]. However, in our practice and contrary to the experience of others we find uptake and acceptance for this method of external expansion amongst our patients thus far has been very limited.

9. Gluteal contouring

Contouring the gluteal area is synonymous with the Brazilian Buttock Lift (BBL). Fat has gained popularity in its use, as a method of adding volume to the gluteal area becoming one of the fastest growing procedures in aesthetic surgery, and it is often performed as an adjunct to body contouring [34]. In 1987, Toledo presented one of the first studies investigating fat transfer in buttock augmentation in the USA [35].

To reduce the risks associated with injecting fat in the buttocks, we inject the fat above the muscle using a 5 mm cannula approaching in an acute angle. This angle of approach makes it more difficult to penetrate the deeper gluteal muscles layer.

When transferring fat to the buttocks, it is of paramount importance to utilise handheld high-definition ultrasound to determine the plane and depth of injection.

In our practice, we do not utilise silicone implants to contour the buttocks as we see fat transfer to be a more practical and safer option when performed by appropriately trained Plastic surgeon/s [36].

In our opinion and the collective opinion of others, fat transfer is the gold standard for gluteal augmentation, as we feel it gives a natural look to the gluteal area with high patient satisfaction [37].

The procedure has been made even safer with the advent of handheld high-definition ultrasound, which gives a visual on the anatomical location, and depth of the transferred fat into the buttocks, thus avoiding the gluteal muscles and reducing risks of embolus and vascular origin complications [38–41].

In our practice, VASER is used when harvesting fat for BBL. BBL is usually the final stage of 360-body contouring. For simplicity of description, we had attributed the terminology the fourth dimension for this combination of surgery (**Figure 10**).

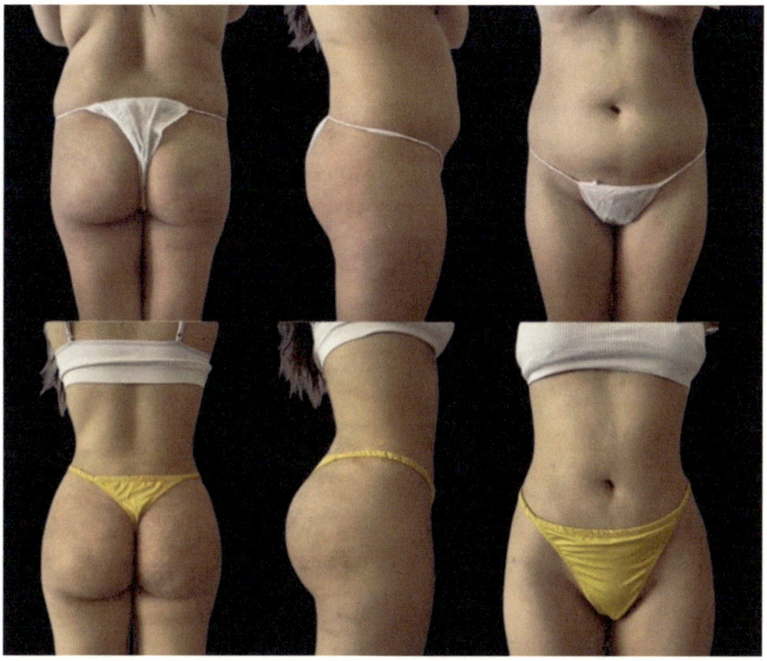

Figure 10.
Twenty-four-year-old female. Six months following VASER 360 liposculpture of abdomen, flanks and back with 800 cc fat transfer each buttock area, Brazilian butt lift (BBL).

The reason of leaving BBL to the end of the sequence of operative procedures is for avoidance of the patient being on her buttocks for the duration of a relatively lengthy surgery, thus avoiding unnecessary pressure on the transferred fat.

10. Patient selection

The criteria of patients' selection for body contouring are unchanged from our last published chapter in Enhanced Liposuction New Perspective and Techniques 2022 [42]. However, when we are considering fat transfer be it for breasts, abdomen or gluteal region, we take into account four criteria.

For the sake of clarity, we have listed these criteria as anatomical structures from the most superficial tissue layer to the deepest.

These criteria include:

1. Skin, quality, laxity, excess and distribution.

2. Fat, deep and superficial, which is below and above Scarpa's fascia, respectively.

3. The deep fascia and muscles.

4. Surface anatomy and relationship with deep structures.

Why is this important to us?

The skin plays a major role in outcomes. For example, if the skin quality is poor, then the skin may need further non-surgical tightening, one example is the use of monopolar radiofrequency. In our practice, we use INDIBA Deep-care as our monopolar radiofrequency device of choice for its ease of use with very low risks and almost non-existent downtime. If the skin has significant excess, then surgical removal is warranted, examples are mastopexy and abdominoplasty.

The liposuction of the deep fat is for the aim of debulking the envelope; however, liposuction of the superficial fat is for sculpturing it to re-create shadows and light reflections to a near perfect body contouring. When adding volume in the relevant space/s, we create the fourth dimension.

11. Patient safety

How do we uphold the highest safety levels when considering patients for body contouring including VASER liposculpture, fat transfer and excisional surgery?

This starts with patient selection and the appropriate surgery in addition to having the relevant instrumentations. Accurate planning is a prerequisite for successful cosmetic surgical outcomes. Precise meticulous execution of the surgical plan is paramount in achieving the best aesthetic outcomes.

Let us not forget in this equation that the surgeon's and team safety is equally as important as the patient. One simple example is the distance the surgeon's arm travels when performing a large volume liposculpturing procedure.

We calculated the distance travelled in 4–5 hours of 360-body contouring procedure could be in the region of 10 miles; however, if the height of the table is adjusted by few centimetres, this could reduce the distance the surgeon/s hand and upper limb travelled by ~25%.

One must remember that a surgeon's journey is 20–25 years in practice, and this type of surgery weighs heavily on his/her joints of the hand and upper limb in addition to the neck. Hence, one must protect the surgeon and the team as they experience the same stresses on their physique during such time intensive surgery with high concentration levels, and the environment must be relaxing and harmonious.

12. Summary

Selecting the right patient for the relevant procedure, using the appropriate instrumentations whilst having the necessary skills and expertise, is of profound importance. Additionally, it is a must to have a well-trained, cohesive team, which functions at the highest levels of governance.

These two factors will further contribute to patients' safety and good surgical aesthetic outcomes, whilst minimising risks and potential complications.

On the one hand, such provision of service must have at its foundation an ethical patient-centred approach.

On the other hand, aspiring to the continuous development of the team involved in the patient journey from the first point of contact and until discharge is of profound importance. This is the ethos on which we have built our practice.

Author details

Ali Juma[1*], Jamil Hayek[2] and Simon Davies[3]

1 Consultant Plastic Surgeon, The Clinic @51, Liverpool, United Kingdom

2 Plastic Surgeon, Hayek Clinic, Kaunas, Lithuania

3 Solta EMEA, Barcelona, Spain

*Address all correspondence to: alijuma@me.com

References

[1] The Cambridge English, E-Dictionary

[2] Rubin P, Jewell ML, Richter D, Uebel CO. Body Contouring and Liposuction. 1st ed. In: Pitanguy I, editor. Introduction. United Kingdom: Elsevier Saunders; 2013. pp. 1-3

[3] Zukowski ML, Ash K. Ultrasound assisted Lipoplasty learning curve. Aesthetic Surgery Journal. 1998;**12**(2):104-110

[4] Troillus C. Ultrasound assisted Lipoplasty is it really safe? Aesthetic Plastic Surgery. 1999;**23**(5):307-311

[5] Jewell ML, Fodor PB, De Souza Pinto EB, Al Shammari MA. Clinical application of VASER-assisted Lipoplasty: A pilot clinical study. Aesthetic Surgery Journal. 2002;**22**:131-146

[6] Hoyos A, Prendergast PM. High-Definition Body Sculpting Art and Advanced Lipoplasty Techniques. Berlin, Heidelberg: Springer-Verlag; 2014. ISBN 978-3-642-54890-1

[7] Hoyos A, Millard JA. VASER-assisted high-definition Liposculpture. Aesthetic Surgery Journal Volume 27, issue 6, November 2007, pages 594-604

[8] Der Meulen V, Richard M. Consideration Generales Sur Les Greffes Graisseues et Serograissuses apiloiques et Leurs principals Applications Paris These. 1919:11

[9] Costanzo D, Romco A, Marena F. Autogenous fat grafting in plastic surgery: An historical perspective. EPlasty. 1 March 2022;**22**:e4

[10] Czerny M. Reconstruction of the breast with a lipoma. Chir Kongr Verh. 1895;**2**(2):216

[11] Brunning P. Contribution a l' etude des greffe adipeuses. Bulletin et Mémoires de l'Académie Royale de Médecine de Belgique. 1919;**28**:220

[12] Fischer A, Fischer G. First surgical treatment for moulding body's cellulite with three 5mm incisions. Bulletin of the International Academy of Cosmetic Surgery. 1976;**3**:35

[13] Colmen SR. Long term survival of fat transplants: Controlled demonstrations. Aesthetic Plastic Surgery. 1995;**19**:421-425

[14] Klein JA. The tumescent technique: Anaesthesia and modified liposuction technique. Dermatologic Clinics. July 1990;**8**(3):425-437

[15] Wu S, Coombs DM, Gurunian R. Liposuction: Concept, safety and techniques in body-contouring surgery. Cleveland. Journal of Medicine. 31 July 2020;**87**(8):476

[16] Wah D, Amirlak B, Rohrich R, Davis K. The clinical importance of the fat compartments in Midfacial aging. Plastic and Reconstructive Surgery. Global Open. 2013;**1**(19):e92

[17] Goisis M, Stella E, Rosset L. Nano fat grafting compared to hyaluronic acid and PRP treatment of the lower lid and tear trough: Clinical outcome. JSM Ophthalmology. 2015;**3**(1):1027

[18] Gonzalez F, Armando E, Chavez P, Francisco M, Guerrero R, Rene O, et al. A new surgical approach to body contouring. PRS Global Open. 2021;**9**(5):e3540

[19] Duscher D, Atashroo D, Maan ZN, Luan A, Brett EA, Barrera J, et al.

Ultrasound-assisted liposuction does not compromise the regenerative potential of adipose-derived stem cells. Stem Cells Translational Medicine. 2016;**5**(2):248-257

[20] Duscher D, Maan ZN, Luan A, Aitzetmüller MM, Brett EA, Atashroo D, et al. Ultrasound-assisted liposuction provides a source for functional adipose-derived stromal cells. Cryotherapy. 2017;**19**(12):1491-1500

[21] Cheriyan T, Kao H-K, Qiao X, Guo L. Low harvest pressure enhances autologous fat graft viability. Plastic and Reconstructive Surgery. 2014;**133**(6):1365-1368

[22] Seaman SA, Tannan ST, Cao Y, Liu KY. Differential effects of processing time duration of collagenase digestion on human and murine fat grafts. Plastic and Reconstructive Surgery. 2015;**136**(2):189e-199e

[23] Ian C, Hanwright Philip J, Gutowski Karol A, Kim John Y. Is there a limit? A risk assessment model of liposuction volume on complications in Lipoabdominoplasty. PRS. 2015;**136**(45):92-93

[24] Coleman SR, Saboeiro A. A Primary breast augmentation with fat grafting. Clinics in Plastic Surgery. 2015;**42**(3):301-306 vii

[25] Report on autologous fat transplantation. ASPRS ad-hoc committee on new procedures. Plastic Surgical Nursing. 1987;7(4):140-141

[26] Leong DT, Hutmacher DW, Chew F, Lim TC. Procedure applications and outcomes of autologous fat grafting. Annals of Medicine and Surgery. 2017;**20**:49-60

[27] Gutowski KA, ASPS Fat Graft Task Force. Current applications and safety of autologous fat grafts: A report of the ASPS fat graft task force. Plastic and Reconstructive Surgery. 2009;**124**(01):272-280

[28] Mathew J. Davis et al, application of fat grafting in cosmetic breast surgery. Seminars in Plastic Surgery. 2020;**34**(1):24-29

[29] Pu LL, Coleman SR, Cui X, Ferguson RE, Jr VHC. Autologous fat grafts harvested and refined by the Coleman technique: A comparative study. Plastic and Reconstructive Surgery. 2008;**122**(03):932-937

[30] Erdim M, Tezel E, Numanoglu A, Sav A. The effects of the size of liposuction cannula on adipocyte survival and the optimum temperature for fat graft storage: An experimental study. Journal of Plastic, Reconstructive & Aesthetic Surgery. 2009;**62**:1210-1214

[31] Kakagia D, Pallua N. Autologous fat grafting: in search of the optimal technique. Surgical Innovation. 2014;**21**(03):327-336

[32] Skillman J, McManus P, Bhaskar P, Hamilton S, Roy PG, O'Donoghue JM. UK guidelines for lipomodelling of the breast on behalf of plastic, reconstructive & aesthetic surgery & association of breast surgery expert advisory group. JPRAS. Feb 2022;**75**(2):511-518

[33] Khouri R, Eisenmann-Klein M, Cardoso E, Cooley BC, Gombos E, Baker TJ. Brava and autogenous fat transfer is a safe & effective breast augmentation alternative: Results of a 6 years 81-patients prospective multi-centre study. Plastic and Reconstructive Surgery. 2021;**129**(5):1173-1187

[34] Wong A, Alexander BS, Selsky DJ, Zuriarain A. Safety of wireless ultrasound–guided gluteal fat grafting. The American Journal of Cosmetic Surgery. Marc 2021;**38**(1):21-23

[35] Toledo LS. Gluteal augmentation with fat grafting: The Brazilian buttock technique: 30 years' experience. Clinics in Plastic Surgery. 2015;**42**(02):253-261

[36] Rios L, Gupta V. Improvement in Brazilian butt lift (BBL) safety with the current recommendations from ASERF, ASAPS, ISAPS. Aesthetic Surgery Journal. 13 July 2020;**40**(8):864-870

[37] O'Neill RC, Abu-Ghname A, Davis MJ, Chamata E, Ramos CK, Winocour SJ. The role of fat grafting in buttock augmentation. Seminars in Plastic Surgery. 2020;**34**(1):38-46

[38] Del Vecchio D, Kenkel JM. Practice advisory on gluteal fat grafting. Aesthetic Surgery Journal. 24 Aug 2022;**42**(9):1019-1029

[39] Rios LM. Commentary on: Practice advisory on gluteal fat grafting. Aesthetic Surgery Journal. 24 Aug 2022;**42**(9):1030-1031

[40] Tillo O, Nassab R, Pacifico M. BAAPS Gluteal Fat Grafting Safety Review- and Recommendation. 30th September 2022

[41] Statement of Patient Safety During Gluteal Fat Grafting Endorsed By The International Society For Aesthetic Plastic Surgery (ISAPS), American Society of Plastic Surgeons (ASPS), The Plastic Surgery Foundation (PSF), The Aesthetic Society and Aesthetic Surgery Education and Research Foundation (ASERF). 26 October 2022

[42] Juma A, Hayek J, Davies S. The safe evolution of liposuction into Liposculpture. In: Enhanced Liposuction New Perspective and Techniques. London, UK, London, UK: 5772/ intechopen; 2022. pp. 17-28 91537

Section 3

Surgical Body Contouring

Chapter 4

Perspective Chapter: Gluteal Augmentation with Complete Retromuscular Placement of Biconvex Silicone Implants

Valerio Badiali, André Salval and Salvatore Giordano

Abstract

Permanent esthetic buttocks augmentation is on the rise. Fat augmentation or Brazilian butt lift (BBL) cannot be a solution for patient with a lean body and poor subcutaneous fat deposit. Hyaluronic acid (HA) infiltrations for volume enhancement, when used in big volumes, tend to form foreign body granulomas and cysts, which are visible and palpable with a poor esthetic result. On the other hand, implant-based augmentations have been proposed since the late 1960 of the past century. Buttocks implants can be placed in four different planes according to distinct surgical techniques: subcutaneous, subfascial, intramuscular, and submuscular. An alternative to the widely proposed intramuscular technique is described in the chapter. Submuscular positioning of a biconvex silicone implant is a safe and valuable alternative to other gluteal augmentation techniques with a different plane for implant positioning. Depending on implant volume, submuscular gluteal augmentation has the benefit to perfectly conceal the implant making it almost impalpable and invisible as well.

Keywords: gluteal implant augmentation, retromuscolar, buttocks implants, gluteoplasty, biconvex silicone implants

1. Introduction

Gluteoplasty with implants is a growing trend within surgical esthetic procedures. Endpoint of the procedure is enhancement of the roundness of buttocks, volume augmentation along with outward projection. Permanent and stable results are obtainable only with fat grafting and/or gluteal implants placement. Patients with a lean body and low gluteal projection have no choice but to undergo gluteal implant surgery, since conspicuous donor areas are needed for fat grafting. Gluteal implants may be sufficient or can even be associated with fat transfer in a combined procedure [1]. Techniques for implant-based buttocks augmentation are divided into subcutaneous, subfascial, intramuscular, and submuscular, according to the depth of the plane in which the implant pocket is made. The gluteus maximus muscle can be uplifted to expose the "subgluteal

IntechOpen

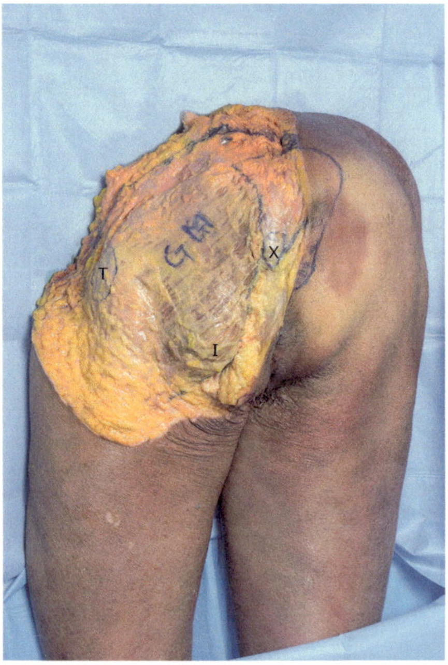

Figure 1.
Skin and subcutaneous tissue have been removed to show the superficial anatomy of the gluteal region. Palpable landmarks are coccyx (X) greater trocanther (T) and Ischial tuberosity (I). Gluteus maximus fibers run diagonally from the origin (lateral margin of sacral bone and coccyx) and insert into the iliotibial band and on the gluteal tuberosity.

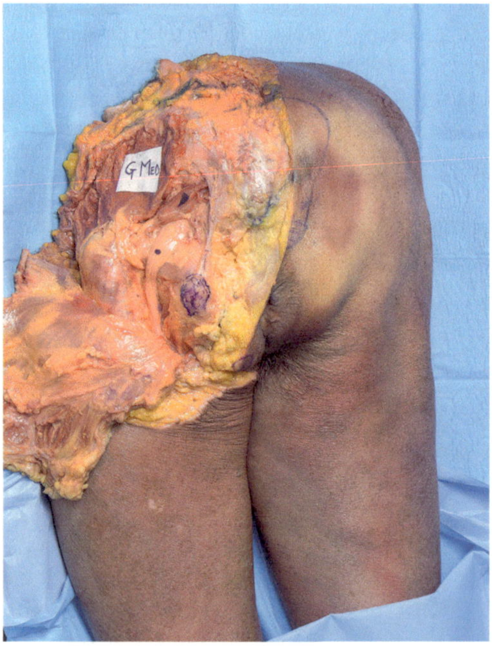

Figure 2.
Gluteus maximus has been elevated and detached from his origin from sacral bone and coccyx. Deep face of implant pocket may be seen, with piriformis muscle (blue triangle) and ischiatic nerve (blue dot). G Med: gluteus medius.

cellular space," as described by Robles et al. in 1984 [2]. To better understand the anatomy of the gluteal region, a cadaveric dissection was made by second author (A.S.). Ischial tuberosity is an important landmark for the surgery planification, along with sacrotuberous ligament; both structures delimit the medial border of the implant pocket, in order avoid dissection into the ischioanal space. The deep face of the pocket is represented by muscle piriformis, superior and inferior gemelli, internus and externus obturator, and quadratus femoris. Ischiatic nerve origin is just below piriformis muscle in more than 85% of the population [3]. **Figure 1** shows superficial anatomy of the gluteal region. **Figure 2** depicts relevant anatomy of the deep gluteal region.

2. The retromuscolar technique for implant-based gluteal augmentation

Complications of every gluteal implant-based surgery such as seroma formation, wound dehiscence, implant extrusion, and/or implant visibility and palpability can be greatly reduced with the choice of a submuscular placement of the implant [4–6]. Advantages of this surgical technique are short length of skin incisions, very low rate of implant exposure or extrusion, short operative time, and full implant concealing, making it much less visible and palpable. Downside may comprehend longer learning curve, blind dissection, and little range of implants size.

Other gluteal augmentation techniques may have an highest rate of complications: implant is visible and palpable when placed in a subfascial plane, especially in patient with a thin subcutaneous layer; poor covering of the implant may lead over time to fat lamination and skin loosening with infragluteal fold displacement [7] and implant dislocation. When the implant is placed in a intramuscular pocket, advantage is better concealing, but still there's a moderate percentage of dislocation due to gluteal muscle contraction [8, 9], disadvantage is muscle atrophy and even longer learning curve. Submuscular undermining in first cases could be an intramuscular dissection, for the fear of damaging the deeper structures. Is such cases, one must remember the anatomy and the fact that he/she's not using any sharp dissection, so damaging structures while creating the pocket is seldom a possibility. Perfect dissection should be performed in a deep plane (under gluteus maximus muscles) with great safety for the sciatic nerve.

3. Patient selection

The retromuscolar technique is preferred by patients requesting a natural, sporty result. Both volume and projection of the buttocks may be improved. Patient with skin laxity of the gluteal area must be carefully advised that little change of this problem will be achieved, especially at the level of infragluteal fold.

Preoperative indications include patients with minimal gluteal flaccidity and a good gluteal muscle tone. Poor candidates may be patients with spinal disk hernia-tion, sciatic nerve pain and thus should not undergo this kind of gluteal augmentation technique.

4. Technique description

Implant selection must be chosen along with patient desires, but first and foremost by carefully palpating muscle thickness, volume, and tension at the gluteal midpoint area; the first two are essential to understanding what will be the gluteus maximus muscular implant coverage. Authors-preferred implants are biconvex implants from the French company Sebbin. Those implants are filled with a very high cohesive gel. Implant size range is quite narrow at the moment, presenting sizes of 370, 410, 480, and 530 cc. It is preferred to use an implant size ranging from 370 to 410 cc if the muscle is very thin or the patient has a narrow hip circumference.

Higher size from 410 to 480 cc should be used if the muscle has regular thickness or if the patient has a higher hip circumference. Drawing starts with the patient in the standup position (**Figure 3**). A horizontal line is drawn at the top of the intergluteal fold, since this feature will disappear when the patient is in prone position, thus ensuring that the incisions will be made entirely within the intergluteal crease to conceal the final scar. Subsequently, bone landmarks are identified to define the limits of the implant diameter. Those are the trochanter posterior border, i.e., the implant pocket lateral limit.

Another point of reference is the ischial tuberosity; from this point the sacro-tuberous ligament runs toward the sacrum and the course of the lower limit of the gluteal muscle: this is the pocket inferior and medial limit. After drawing the point of desired maximum projection in which we want to place the implant, we obtained the radius of the implant according to implant diameter. Skin incision lines are then drawn with the patient laying over the operating table (**Figure 4**) placing them 1 cm lateral to the midline, with intergluteal fold and sacrodermal ligament complete preservation. Skin incisions are parallel and a little offset to lower the size of the area in between; length is 3–5 cm according to experience of the surgeon and implant choice of size.

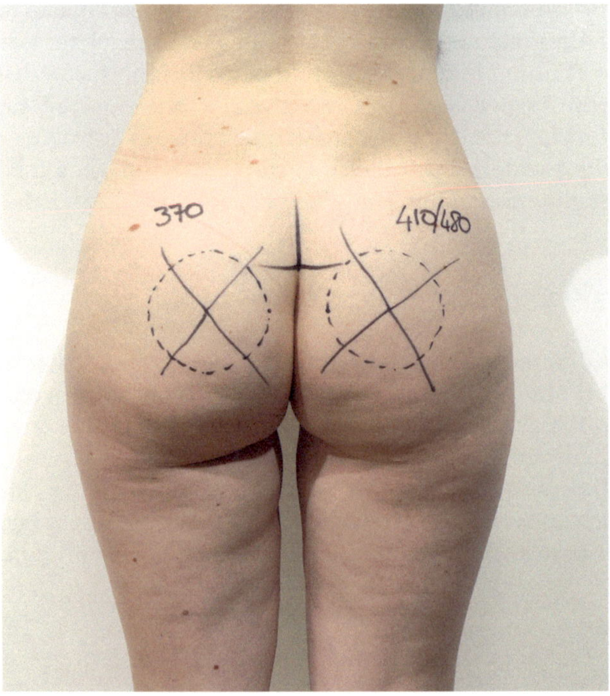

Figure 3.
Drawing in the standing position, horizontal line at the top of intergluteal crease and point of maximum projection of each buttock.

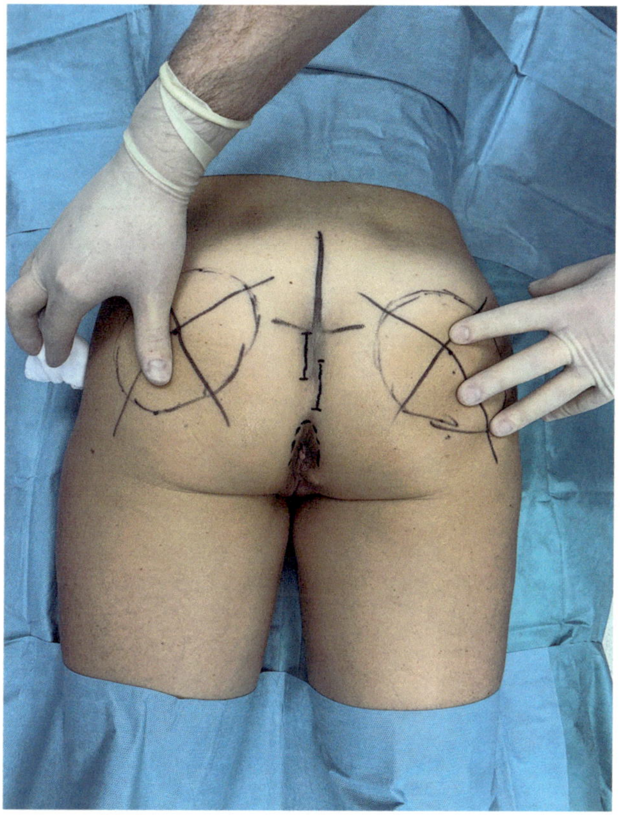

Figure 4.
Drawing in the prone position, offset of skin incision, 3–4 cm long, parallel, and 1 cm lateral to the midline. Skin around the anal region is highlighted in order to avoid incision in that area.

Anesthesia can be general, deep sedation, or even spinal. We do not prefer the latter due to the fact of dilation of the vein system that could lead to a higher chance of bleeding. Patient decubitus is prone and completely flat. Incision lines are then drawn as described above and infiltrated with analgesic solution (2 mg epinephrine and 20 ml of ropivacaine 7.5 mg/ml for every 1000 ml of saline). This solution is infiltrated under the incision lines dermis, in the full thickness of subcutaneous fat and the medial border of gluteus maximus fascia; total volume is around 50 ml on each side. After that one must take time to wait for the drug onset, around 10–20 minute. Then a stab incision is made with a 15-scalpel blade in the middle of incision lines, a 2.5 mm infiltration cannula is inserted, and the submuscular plane is infiltrated with the same solution. This step is very important for the upcoming procedure of pocket dissection. The cannula must first pierce the gluteus maximus fascia (a perforating sound might be heard), then moved 2 cm deeper, and then turned laterally, to infiltrate the solution deeper to the gluteus maximus muscle, in the space between gluteus maximus and piriformis medially and between gluteus maximus and gluteus medius laterally. A first-time error could be a too superficial infiltration. Subsequently, time is taken to allow epinephrine to exert its vasoconstrictive effect. After scrubbing the skin with chlorhexidine and alcohol solution and sterile draping, a sterile gauze is tapered over the anal region to isolate it. The instruments required for submuscular gluteal augmentation have been designed by Petit F as described in his paper [9]. Those are a mayo scissors, a Colin Hartman retractor, two long spacers (**Figure 5**), forceps, and a disposable funnel for implant insertion. No diathermic cutting instruments or bipolar forceps are routinely used. After the skin incision, opening continues bluntly in the subcutaneous tissue with the scissors to reach the insertion of gluteus maximus at the lateral border of the sacrum. In this, dissection is limited in the subcutaneous region and over the muscular fascia to keep at a minimum the dead space formation. After that muscolar fascia is perforated with the closed scissors, and this tiny hole is enlarged by the opening of the instrument while regressing it. Then the surgeon's index finger can access the submuscular cellular space. At this point, the surgeon should maintain the depth of the plane of undermining, which is performed bluntly by the fingers with a sweeping motion. Care is taken to maintain the undermining superior and lateral to the sacro-tuberous ligament, thus avoiding the posterior aspect of the obturator foramen. After creating a small cavity by fingers, the long spacers are used to free the pocket from the strongest fascial adhesions. A dry laparotomic gauze is then placed into it, to keep it wide open and to check for major bleedings. Same procedure is then done on the contralateral side, checking for pocket symmetry. With this technique

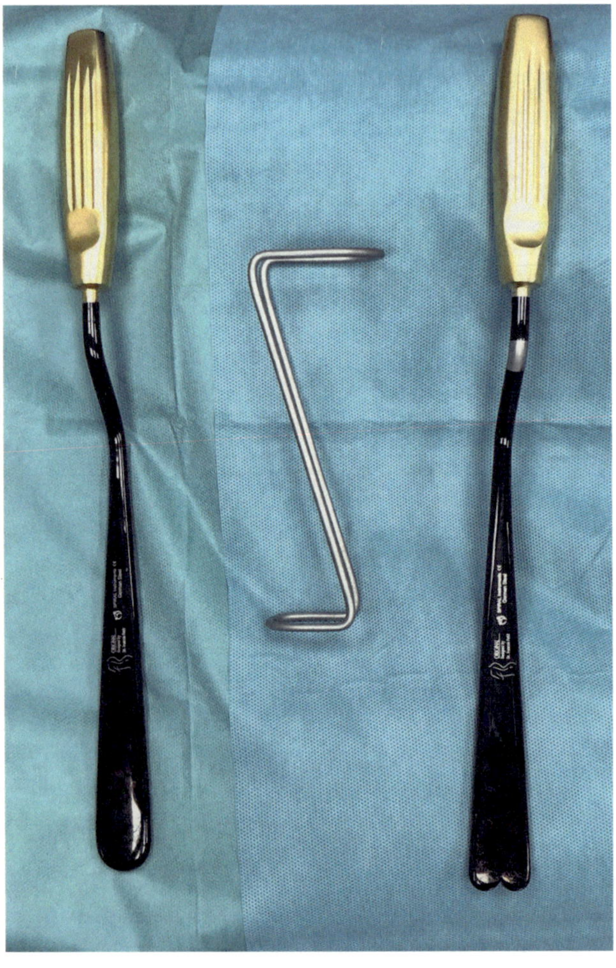

Figure 5.
Surgical instruments needed for pocket dissection and implant placement.

the sciatic nerve is respected in its integrity because the narrow tunnel is made with fingers only as far as the fingers may undermine the muscle and open the pocket. This submuscular elevation allows the entire thickness of the muscle to be elevated, ensuring that the implant will be covered by the full thickness of the muscle. Thus, muscle fibers' morbidity is much less when compared to the one observed in the intramuscular technique. The implant will rest in a deep pocket with little chance of extrusion since muscle contraction will indeed force it to stay in its location. We should remind that

Postoperative complications (in order of frequency)
Wound Dehiscence
Sciatic pain (more than 10 days postoperative)
Wound skin border superficial necrosis
Wound Dehiscence with infection and atb treatment
Asymmetry in implant pocket placement

Table 1.
Specific complication in order of frequency.

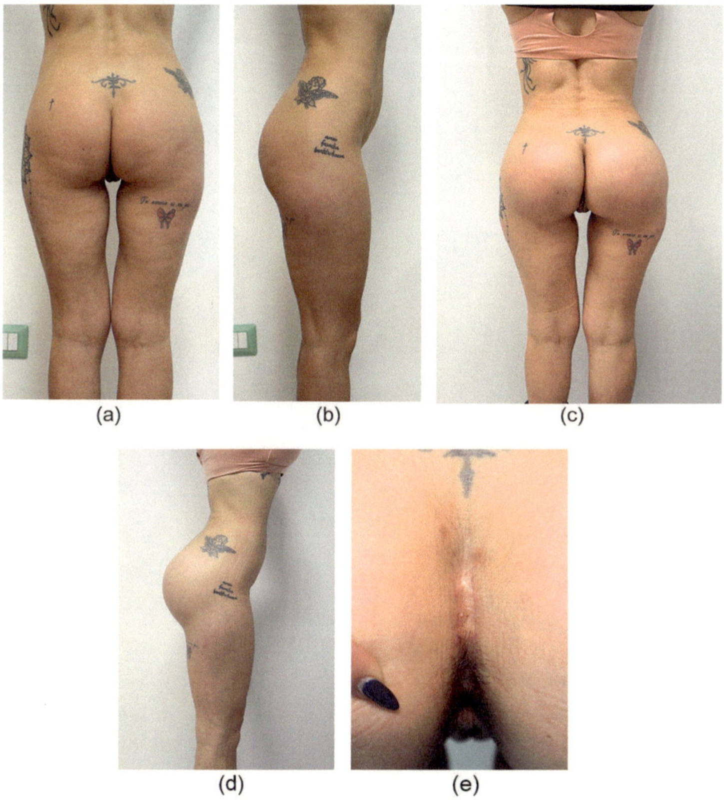

Figure 6.
(a) Preoperative posterior view of 38-year-old female patient. A 480 cc implant placement was planned. (b) Preoperative lateral view of. (c) postoperative posterior view. 3 month postop. (d) Postoperative lateral view. 3 month postop. (e) Close-up of scar placement and quality of patient shown in this figure.

no sharp dissection is used in this surgical technique: Tissues are expanded: fascia and muscle are not cut, but once the tunnel is created, the tissues are dilated progressively. The disposable funnel allows insertion of the implant through the short skin incision and narrow muscular tunnel. Drains are not routinely used. The fascial opening is left untouched, and skin closure is performed in two layers: deep subcutaneous is brought together with a long, ½ circle needle, on a 2–0 braided absorbable suture, then a 3–0 absorbable monofilament close to the dermal plane, by a running bottom to top intradermal suture. The patient is allowed to stand up after being positioned in a supine position for 1 hour and then walk and sit with little restrictions for the first week postoperative. Patients are routinely discharged a few hours after surgery and go back home with a low waist elastic compression garment.

Oral therapy for pain control consists of paracetamol 500 mg/codeine 30 mg bid and ketorolac oral drops along with a muscle relaxant such as diazepam. Steroids may be administered later in case of sciatic nerve irritation. Physical activity (i.e., gym

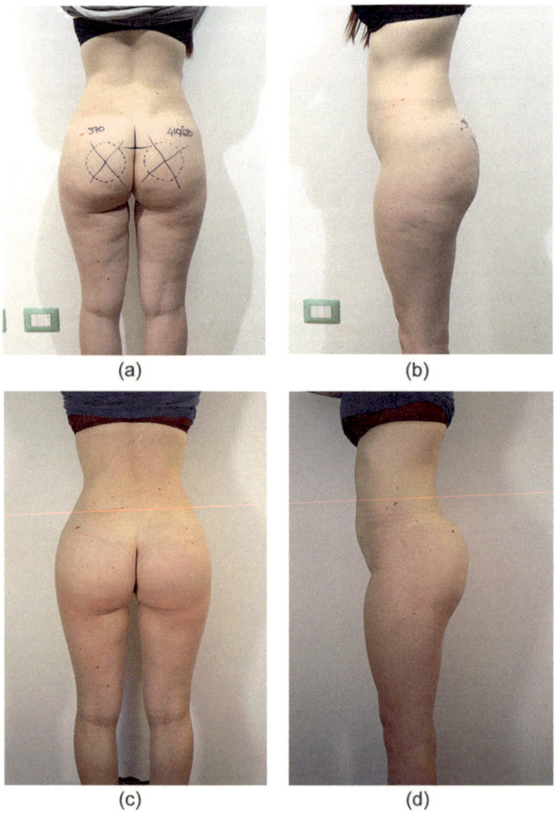

Figure 7.
(a) Preoperative posterior view of 31-year-old female patient. A 370 cc on the left side and a 410 on the right side cc implant placement was planned. (b) Preoperative lateral view. (c) Postoperative posterior view. 4 month postop. (d) Postoperative lateral view. 4 month postop.

workout and any other sport) is discontinued for 4 weeks after surgery. The first outpatient control is 7 days after surgery. The dressing pad is removed, and the incision site is cleaned with antiseptic solution.

Immediate and late complications are listed in **Table 1**.

Cases photography are shown in **Figures 6–10**.

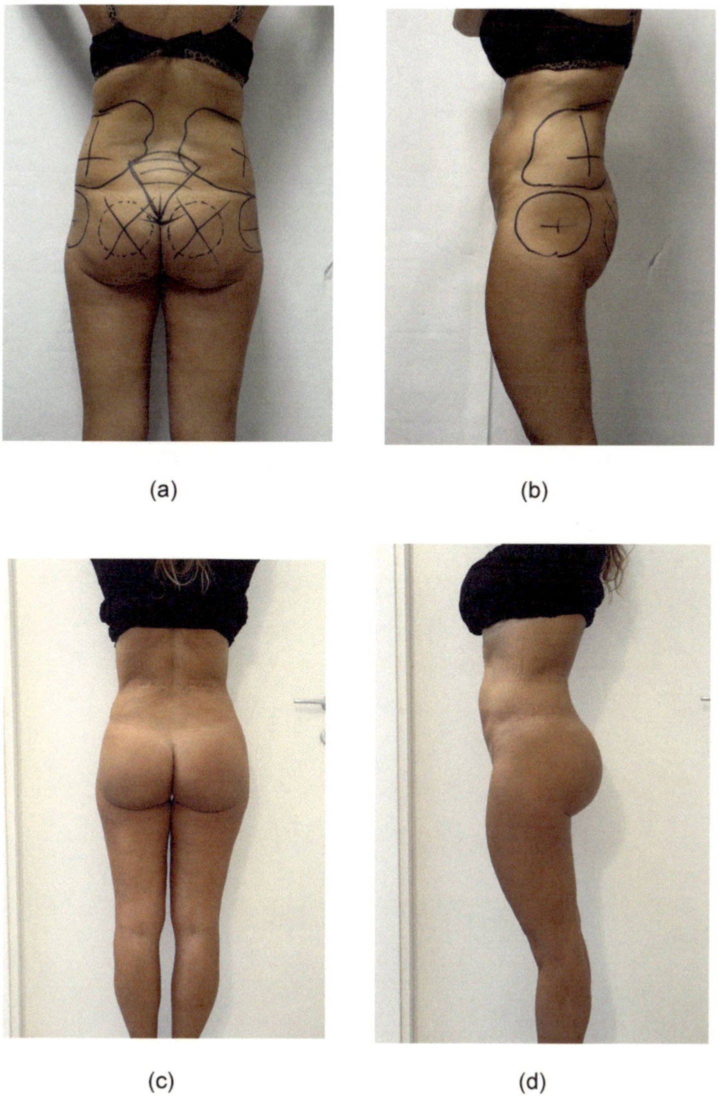

Figure 8.
(a) Preoperative posterior view 52-year-old female patient. A 480 cc implant placement was planned, along with liposuction of flanks and lipofilling of lateral depressed gluteal region (hybrid gluteoplasty). (b) Preoperative lateral view. (c) Postoperative posterior view. 4 month postop. (d) Postoperative lateral view. 4 month postop.

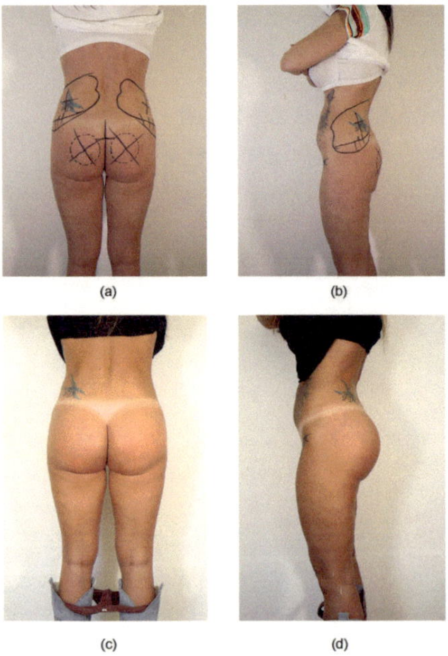

Figure 9.
(a) Preoperative posterior view 53-year-old female patient. A 480 cc implant placement was planned, along with liposuction of flanks. (b) Preoperative lateral view. (c) Postoperative posterior view. 3 month postop. (d) Postoperative lateral view. 3 month postop.

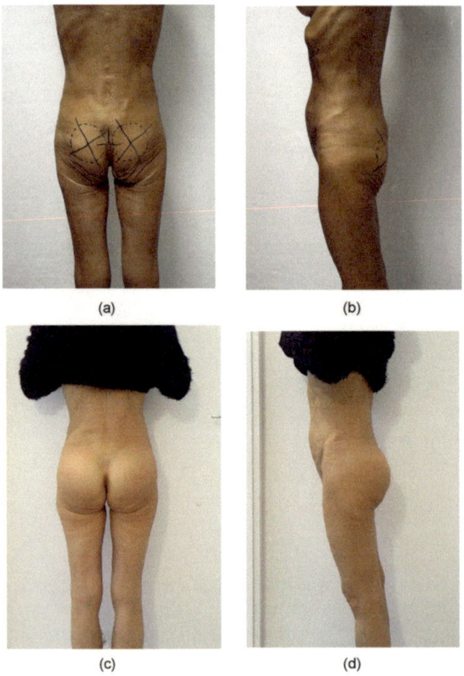

Figure 10.
(a) Preoperative posterior view 51-year-old female patient. A 370 cc implant placement was planned. Patient had a severe laxity of gluteal skin. (b) Preoperative lateral view. (c) Postoperative posterior view. 5 month postop. Improved skin laxity, with residual laxity at the inferior gluteal fold. (d) Postoperative lateral view. 5 month postop.

5. Conclusions

Due to retromuscular plane positioning, implants are invisible in every position of the buttock's region and almost impalpable, giving no clues that the operation was performed, for a natural **esthetic** result. Implant-based gluteal augmentation has a long surgical history, which started back in the late 1960s [1]. Intramuscular placement of the implant has gained popularity over time when compared with the subfascial and subcutaneous plane as it seemed to be the perfect "halfway" between deep and superficial placement [10, 11]. The submuscular placement had less appeal to surgeons for fear of damaging deep structures such as the sciatic nerve or gluteal vessels. This wasn't the case in our experience: sciatic pain is a postoperative complication that can manifest up to 3 week postoperatively, treatment includes oral steroid therapy for 10 days and common pain-controlling drugs. The submuscular technique for gluteal augmentation leads to advantages for both patients and surgeons. Patients seeking a more natural appearance are best candidates for this procedure. Surgeons can perform this technique in a short operative time and without complex preoperative analysis. Great care must be given to the surgical instruments and to the digital undermining, to avoid any damage to the sciatic nerve and the gluteal vessels.

Conflict of interest

The authors declare no conflict of interest.

Author details

Valerio Badiali[1], André Salval[1*] and Salvatore Giordano[2]

1 Istituto Estetico Italiano IEI, Private Practice, Roma, Italy

2 Department of Plastic and General Surgery, Turku University Hospital, Turku, Finland

*Address all correspondence to: a.salval@istitutoesteticoitaliano.it

References

[1] Oranges CM, Tremp M, di Summa PG, et al. Gluteal augmentation techniques: A comprehensive literature review. Aesthetic Surgery Journal. 2017;**37**:560-569

[2] Robles JM, Tagliapietra JC, Grandi MA. Gluteoplastia de aumento: Implante submuscular. Cirugia Plastica Ibero-Latinoamericana. 1984;**71**:365-375

[3] Kirschner JS, Foye PM, Cole JL. Piriformis syndrome, diagnosis and treatment. Muscle & Nerve. 2009;**40**(1):10-18

[4] Lee JW, Kang MG, Park SS. Secondary gluteal augmentation: Surgical technique and outcomes. Plastic and Reconstructive Surgery. 2018;**141**(6):1371-1382

[5] Flores-Lima G, Eppley BL, Dimas JR, Navarro DE. Surgical pocket location for gluteal implants: A systematic review. Aesthetic Plastic Surgery. 2013;**37**(2):240-245

[6] Petit F, Colli M, Badiali V, Ebaa S, Salval A. Buttocks volume augmentation with submuscular implants: 100 cases series. Plastic and Reconstructive Surgery. 2022;**149**(3):615-622

[7] Asserson DB, Kulinich AG, Orbay H, Sahar DE. Differences in complication rates of gluteoplasty procedures that utilize autologous fat grafting, implants, or local flaps. Annals of Plastic Surgery. 2019;**82**(5S Suppl 4):S342-S344

[8] Senderoff DM. Aesthetic surgery of the buttocks using implants: Practice-based recommendations. Aesthetic Surgery Journal. 2016;**36**(5):559-576

[9] Serra F, Aboudib JH, Marques RG. Intramuscular technique for gluteal augmentation: determination and quantification of muscle atrophy and implant position by computed tomographic scan. Plastic and Reconstructive Surgery. 2013;**131**(2): 253e-259e

[10] Vergara R, Amezcua H. Intramuscular gluteal implants: 15 years' experience. Aesthetic Surgery Journal. Mar 2003;**23**(2):86-91

[11] Vergara R, Marcos M. Intramuscular gluteal implants. Aesthetic Plastic Surgery. 1996;**20**:259-26203

Chapter 5

Perspective Chapter: Breast Reduction with Central Pedicle and Autologous Mesh Dermis – Surgical Tecnique

Armin Rudolph Geisse, Klaus Rudolph Oppliger and Thomas Rudolph Oppliger

Abstract

Looking to improve the esthetic and functional results of the central pedicle technique, we add the dermis mesh shaping and support forming a "central cone" to manage the mammary tissue. The periareolar skin agglomeration searches for a reduction in horizontal submammary scars' size. The purpose of this chapter is to describe this surgical technique (combination of techniques).

Keywords: reduction mammoplasty (RM), central pedicle (CP), dermis mesh (DM), periareolar, nipple-areolar complex (NAC)

1. Introduction

There are multiple techniques of Breast Reduction (BR) [1–3] that look to, alongside reducing the size, achieve a symmetric pleasant looking shape, stable through time with minimal ptosis, minimal scarring, and frequency of complications.

Techniques based on structural support from skin and suture usually end up with ptosis and ample scars, because of the weight of the mammary tissue and the expansion of the skin and scars. Besides that, the mammary cone loses firmness and projection.

The BR technique based on the Central Pedicle (CP) was initially described by Balch in 1981 [4] and popularized by Hester in 1985 [5]. It is a trusted technique since the CP has good irrigation and innervation from the perforating branches of the fourth and fifth intercostal spaces [6], and if a wide base is kept, it will also receive irrigation from the perforating branches of the internal mammarian artery and branches from the lateral thoracic artery [5], allowing to reduce great volumes, achieve better mastopexies, and preserve lactation [7–9].

In this chapter, we will show the combination of two techniques: CP + Mesh of Dermis that produces a stable and well-projected central cone, described by Sampaio Goes in 1996 [10, 11] and Circumferential Periareolar Suture described by Benelli in 1990 [12], which allows reducing the submammary scar. Both of these techniques have been proposed in the literature and used separately. By combining them,

IntechOpen

we pretend to obtain better long-term results in shape, reducing ptosis, and achieving minimal submamarian scarring.

This association of techniques has been applied in patients with mamarian hypertrophy and great ptosis, looking to reach the ever-increasing expectations of the patients [13].

We present here a description of this systematized **surgical technique**, complemented with a series of images.

This technique, as well as all the images shown here, and the results of a series of 300 patients who were intervened with this technique, followed and analyzed before, during, and after the procedure; were first published in the "Cirugía Plástica Ibero Latinoamericana" magazine in March 2021, volume 47, N 1, pages 35–48. Used with permission of the editor.

2. Surgical technique

Delineation: All patients are photographed and delineated standing (**Figure 1**). A circle or oval is drawn around the areola marking the borders of the future skin flap: (on average) infraclavicular 16–18 cms to the middle clavicular line; 8–9 cm to middle sternal line; 6 cm to the inframammary fold, and 10–12 cm to the anterior axillary line (**Figures 1** and **2**) by side. The size of the skin flaps (made of fat and skin tissue) depends on the final size of the planned mammary. The circle's cephalic pole (A) (**Figure 2**) is marked 11–12 cm from the middle sternal line, just like the middle point of the lower pole in the new inframammary fold (D) is marked 1 cm over the original fold. From A 6–10 cm are measured downward, toward the external (B) and internal (C) borders of the circle, since a greater length would produce an increased frequency of wrinkles in the skin around the areola. From points B and C, a triangle with a vertex 1 cm under the middle point between the two points is drawn (**Figure 3**), which corresponds to the future point T (joint point of the scars of the flaps under the areola) (**Figure 4**). The same triangle is drawn in point D (**Figure 2**), which corresponds to future point inverted T (joint point of the scars in the inframammary fold). All measurements are confirmed with the anesthetized patient, in a half-seated position,

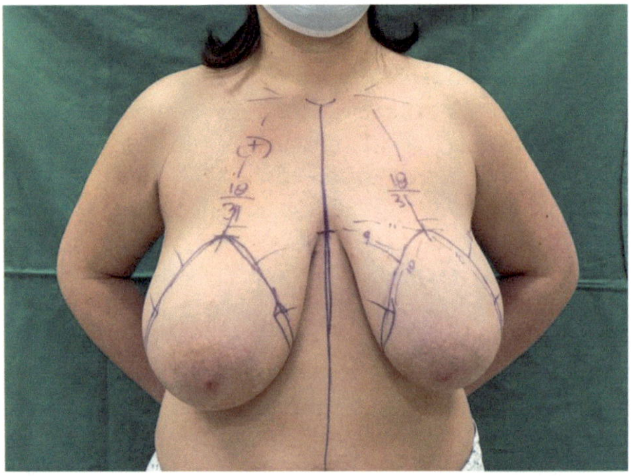

Figure 1.
Photographed and delineated standing.

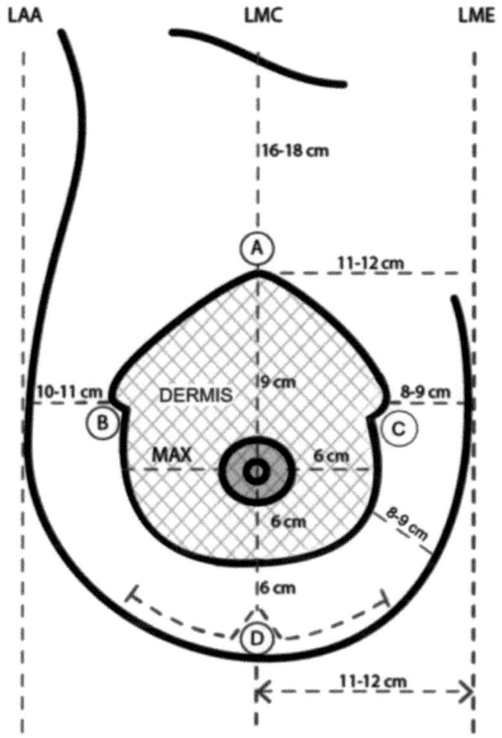

Figure 2.
Preoperative marking scheme [14].

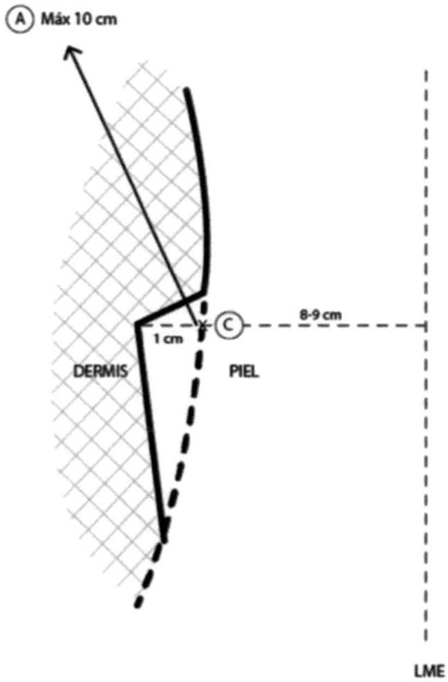

Figure 3.
Skin triangles in B and C (B point is the same as C in the other side of the breast) [14].

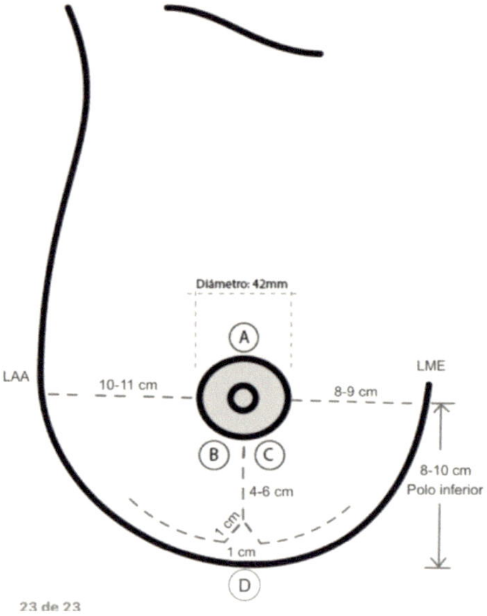

Figure 4.
Final assembly of skin flaps [14].

in the surgical table, utilizing two strings: anchored in the middle line, in the manubrium sternum and xiphoid, for better symmetry.

Surgery: The surgery stars with the subcutaneous infiltration of the mammary, with a saline solution of 240–300cc in each mammary (1.000 cc of physiological saline (PS) + 1 cc of epinephrine +10 cc of sodium bicarbonate (8.4% + 10 ml of lidocaine 2%). We do the marking of the areola with areolotome of 42 mm, and de-epidermize the skin around and until the initially marked circle (**Figure 5**), creating the dermis flaps with a maximum of 9 cm in the cephalic pole, 6 cm toward medial and caudal pole. If the dermis exceeds these measurements, it can be trimmed, but all the

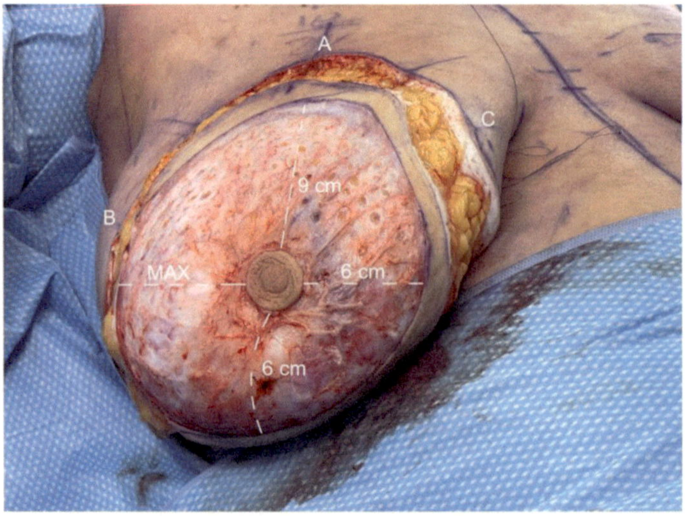

Figure 5.
Measurement of de-epidermised dermis flaps.

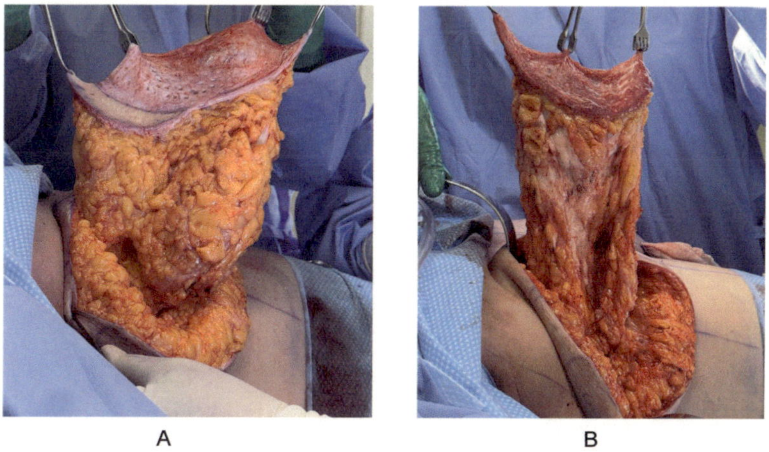

Figure 6.
A. Carved central pedicle (lateral view). B. Central pedicle reduction (lateral view).

lateral dermis must be conserved. The skin-fat flaps are shaped with a bevel cut in the dermis (future periareolar scar) and then, following the superficial fascia of the mammary until the pectoral plane, circumferentially, creating the CP (**Figure 6A**) that is then reduced in four quadrants, slimming it down, and eliminating the excess mammary tissue (under the dermis flaps). More tissue is left under the superior dermis to give it more volume to the future superior pole, and tissue is eliminated in the base as less as possible to conserve irrigation (perforating intercostals of the internal mammary and lateral thoracic arteries), creating a tissue tube or reduced CP (**Figure 6B**). Rigorous hemostasis.

The assembly of the mammary starts with the anchorage of the dermis flaps to the pectoral aponeurosis and/or CP base in all its outline, shaping a mound or central cone (**Figure 7A**) with nylon 4.0 fixing the position of the nipple-areola complex (NAC) (nipple:18–20 cm from the clavicle and 10–11 cm from the middle sternal line). Cuts on the dermis flaps are made to relax it (creating a mesh), and they are extended in order to fix the tension on the mesh, the nipple position, and the shape

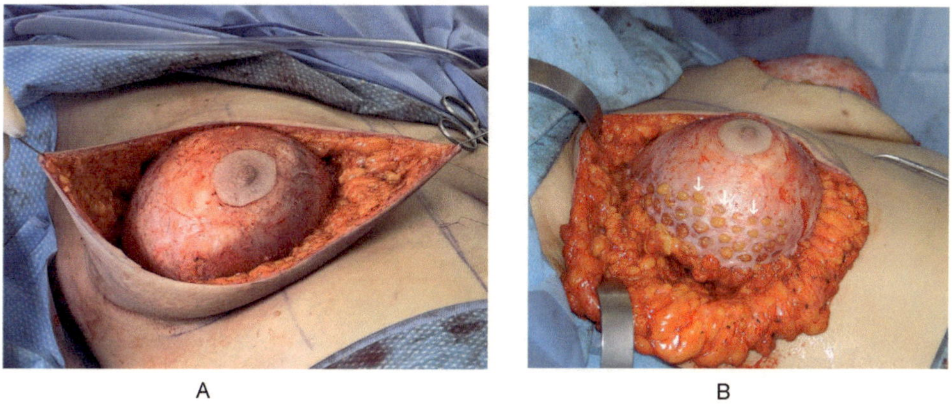

Figure 7.
A. Formation of the mammary cone by suturing the dermis flaps to the pectoral aponeurosis and/or base of the breast. B. Relaxation incisions in the dermis forming a mesh to modify the position of the CAP and reduce the tension of the cone.

of the cone (**Figure 7B**). Once the central mammary cone is done, it is surrounded by the skin flaps creating a double layer, uniting the B and C points of the A-B-C triangle that will contain the areola (**Figures 4** and **8**), Continuous round block on the dermis with polypropylene 3.0 with lancet needle (**Figure 9**), then is tied up calibrating

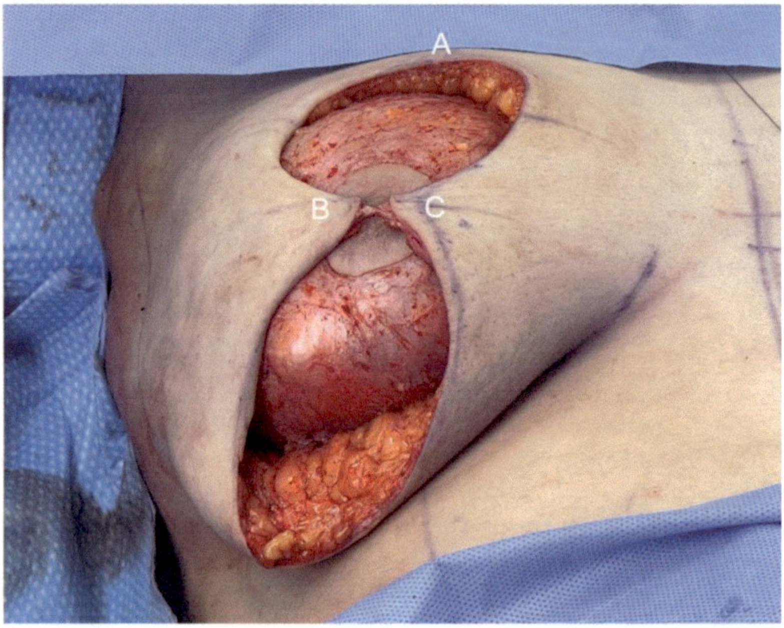

Figure 8.
Suture of points B and C.

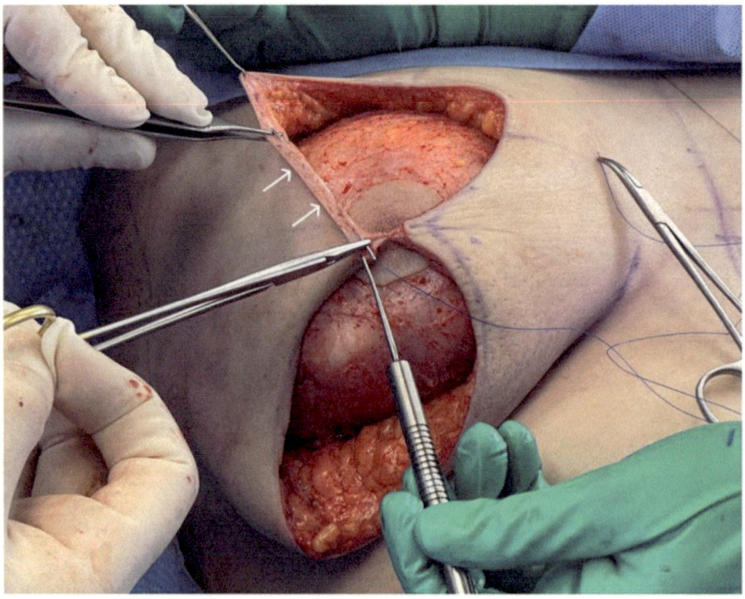

Figure 9.
Start of continuous round block.

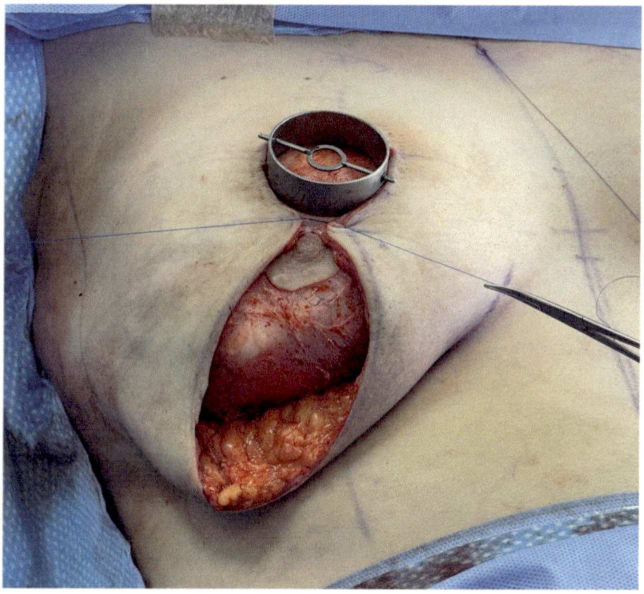

Figure 10.
The knot is anchored to the dermis.

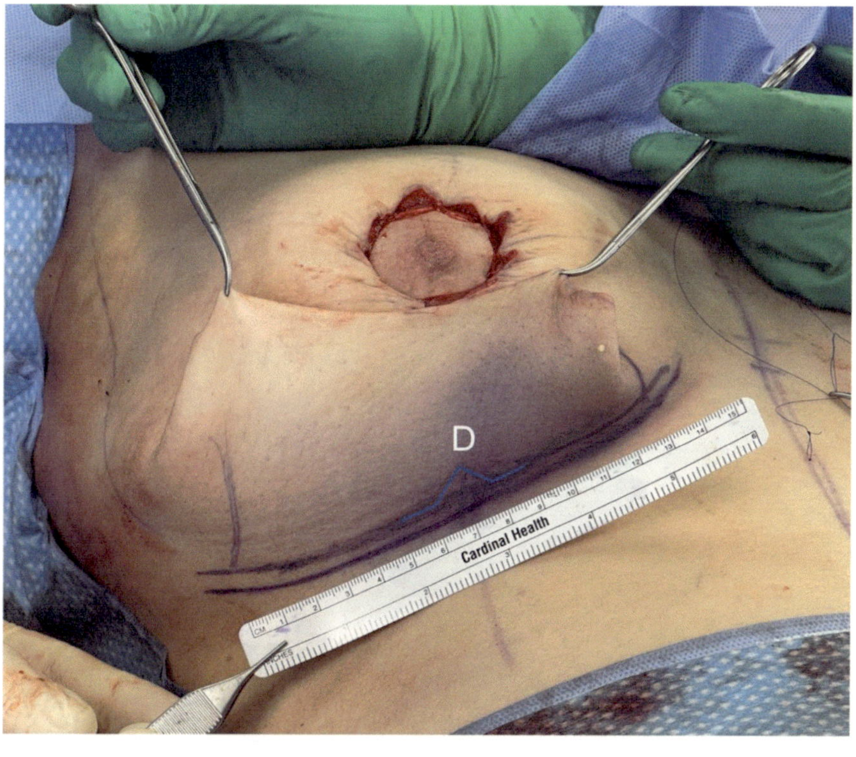

Figure 11.
The inframamary fold.

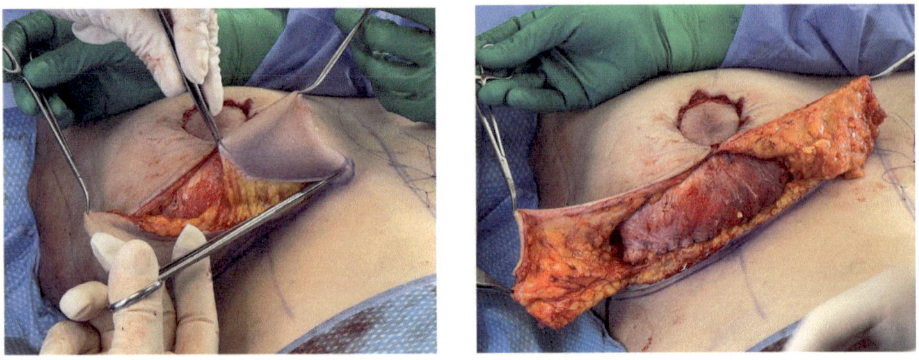

A B

Figure 12.
A. Trimming of inferior pole flaps. B. Extended flaps.

it with the areolotome (**Figure 10**), and the knot is anchored to the dermis of the cone to prevent superficialization (**Figure 10**). The skin is sutured in the two layers: with colorless nylon 5.0 suture on dermis with separate stitches, and the superficial intradermis with nylon 4.0 that is later removed after 14 days of postoperative.

The inframammary fold is marked 1 cm over the original, sculpting the skin triangle of 1 cm in point D (**Figure 11**). The caudal pole's skin flaps are trimmed near the future inframammary fold (**Figure 12A** and **B**), and the superficial fascia of the chest wall is anchored to the dermis of the cone's inferior pole with nylon 4.0, 3.5–4 cm from the bottom edge of the areola, to strengthen the inferior pole (**Figure 13A** and **B**); then, the inferior pole's flaps are pulled towards the lower middle line (**Figure 14A**); they are marked and trimmed leaving 4–5 cm in the middle edge (vertical scar) (**Figure 14B** and **C**).

Two plane sutures of the skin flaps just like the periareolar wound (**Figure 15A–C**). Suction drainage is left in the lateral zone and armpit, which comes out under the inferior pole and is removed 1–2 days before medical discharge. All sutures used are non-resorbable.

For wound care and bandaging, paper tissue is applied as support for the breast for 1 week, until the first wound dressing. The symmetry of the NAC is confirmed

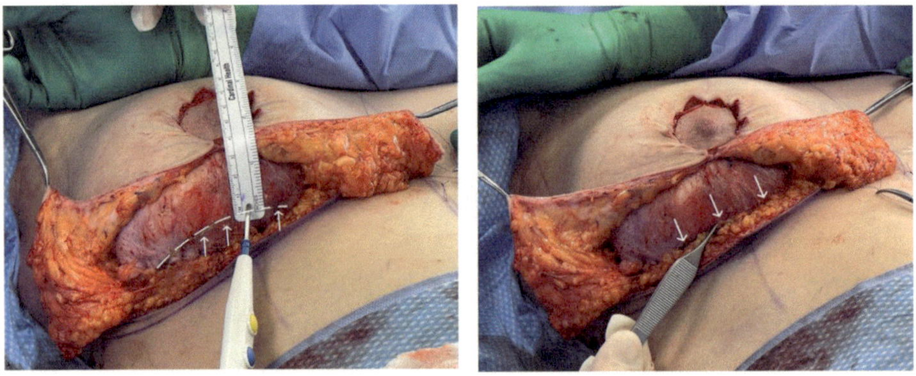

A B

Figure 13.
A–B. Anchorage of Scarpa's fascia to the lower pole of the central mammary cone.

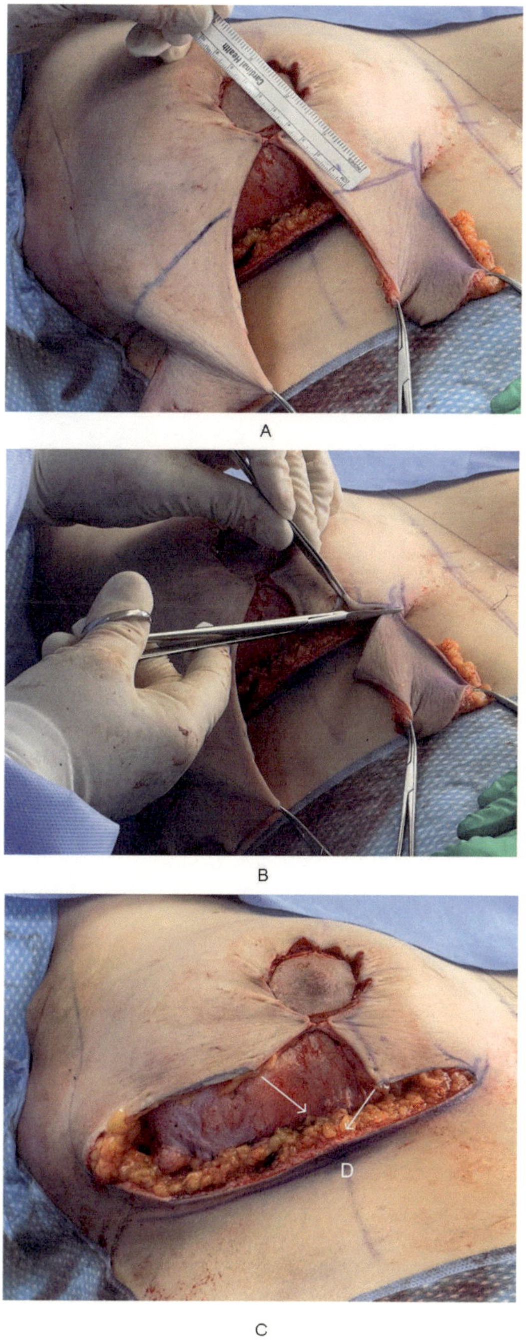

Figure 14.
A and B. C. Definitive carving of lower pole flaps.

with the strings anchored in the middle line (**Figure 16**) during the structuring of the mammaries.

At the end of this work, clinical cases are attached with the aim of demonstrating the results of the described technique (**Figures 17–19**).

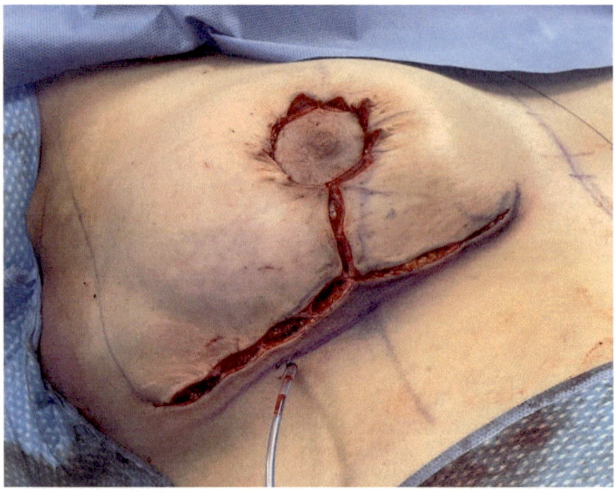

A

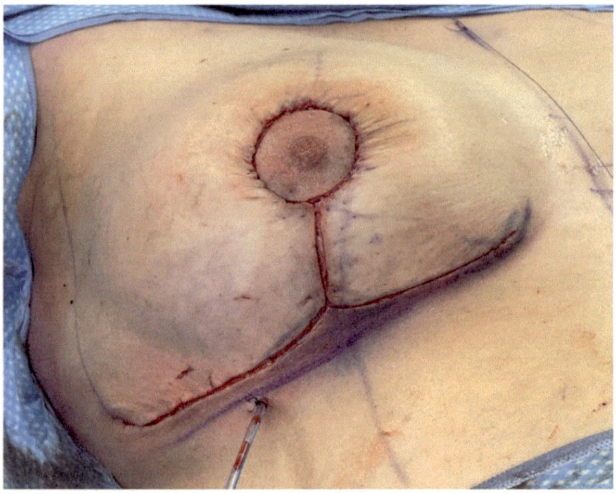

B

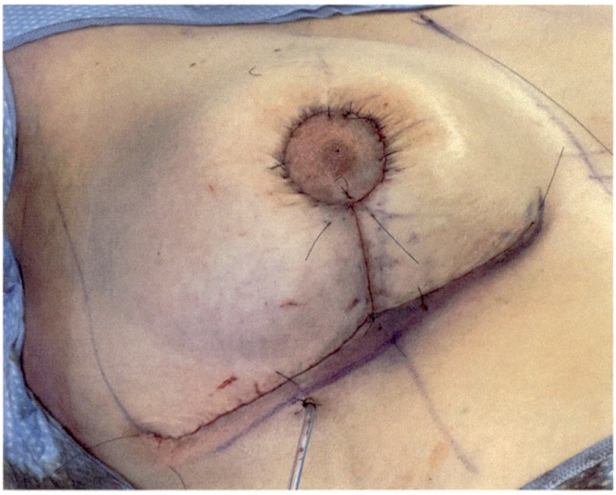

C

Figure 15.
A. Initial suture of dermis. B. Complete suture of dermis. C. Final intradermic suture.

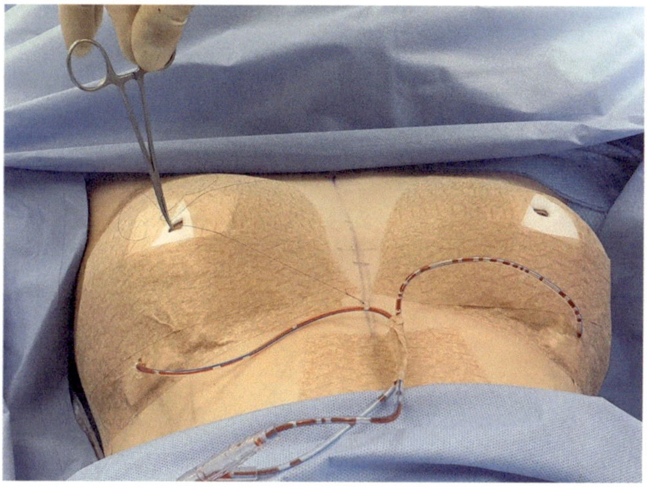

Figure 16.
First wound dressing.

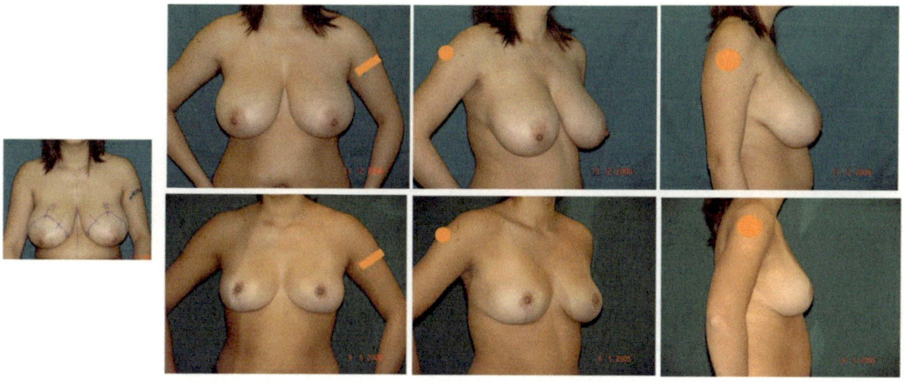

Figure 17.
A case example: the three upper images are before surgery, the lower ones are post-surgery (left image is during demarcation).

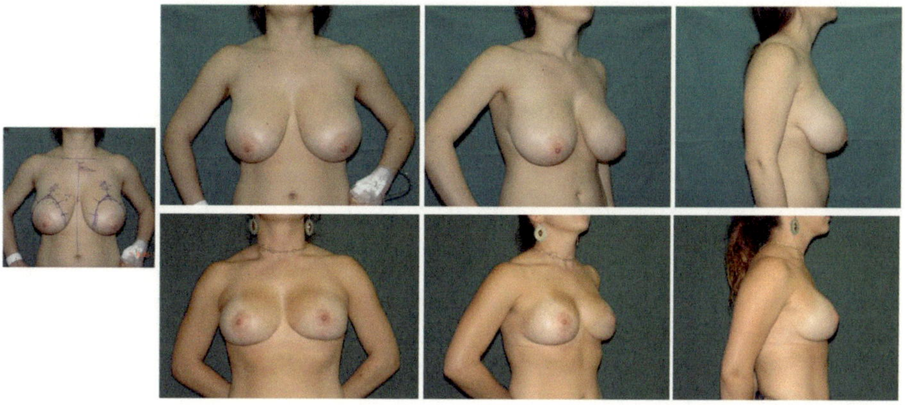

Figure 18.
A second case example.

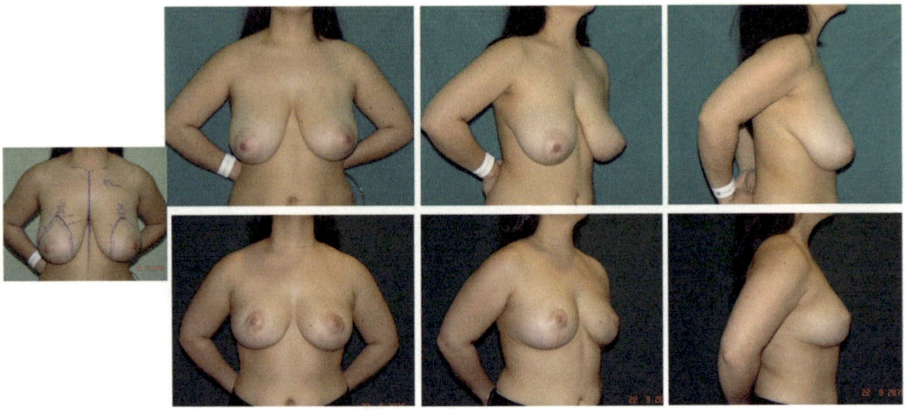

Figure 19.
A third case example.

3. Discussion

When analyzing the traditional techniques of breast reduction, in which the assembling of the reduced pedicles and positioning of the tissues depend on the skin flaps sutured to each other [1–3] and it is them which support the shape and weight of the breast, we tend to see how, in many cases, the weight causes the skin to stretch, the scar to widen, and in the medium and long term we end up seeing breast ptosis, both of the ANP and the inferior pole, causing the breasts to lose shape and firmness.

The combined technique presented here is based on the CP technique (described by Bach [4]) that is safe for removing great volumes and pexies [4–10]. It allows us to: with the dermis mesh (technique described by Góes [11, 12]) that surrounds the CP, one anchored to the aponeurosis creates a stable central cone or mound [10], as a nucleus for the future breast, that in its vertex including the projected and positioned NAC. The reinforcement of the inferior pole of the dermis cone, with the Scarpa fascia suture in its lower third (author's contribution), would reduce the ptosis of the inferior pole. After that, this dermis cone is covered by the skin flaps (double layer), which, with a small tension, help in the firmness of the reduced breast. Suturing around the areola in "Raund Block" described by Benelli [13], accumulating skin around the areola, allows to reduce the inferior horizontal scar, in order to keep it inside the margins of the breast, achieving an average of 13,4 cm in the right breast and 13,2 cm in the left (6,5 to 18 cm), although it is not enough to talk about reduced scarring in all the cases, particularly in big reductions [15]. By cutting the skin 1 cm above the original submammary fold (**Figure 10**), the scar is left in the inferior pole, the compression with silicone becomes easier, and its trauma by the breast holder in the postoperative is prevented. A breast that is firm, pleasant-looking, well projected, round, and stable with minimal ptosis is achieved; just like it was confirmed in the follow-up of the patients and the measurements taken of the nipple to the collarbone and to the submammary fold.

Another difficulty is obtaining adequate breast symmetry at the end of the surgery. This technique allows us to confirm breast symmetry in three stages by comparing the volume of the tissues:

1. When finishing reduces the central pedicles (pulled) and the skin flaps (**Figure 6**).

2. Once the central cone is formed (**Figure 7**). The symmetric position of the NAC is also verified.

3. When the central cone is covered with the skin flaps (**Figure 8**), verify the thickness of the fat-skin flaps, suturing them around the NAC and presenting them when covering the cone.

This achieves an adequate symmetry in 97% of the cases according to questionnaire done to the patients during the postoperative period [14]. Of these patients, 57.7% evaluated the results as "very satisfactory" and 37.9% as "satisfactory."

In all these stages, tissue can be removed if it is necessary for the final symmetry.

In the published series of 300 patients [14], a low frequency of complications is reported (11.3%): re-intervened hematomas (1%), localized hematomas treated by deferred punction (1.3%), total necrosis of the NAC (0.3%), partial necrosis of the NAC (1.3%), necrosis of the skin flap ends greater than 1 cm (2%), fat necrosis greater than 2 cms (2%), hypoesthesia of the NAC (3.3%). All of these are among average or below average frequency of complications described in other techniques [16–21].

In the same series [14], 14.3% of the patients required a surgical touch-up: lateral breast liposuction (7.7%), lipoinjection (1%), scar correction (3%), escharotomies and re-sutures of the skin flaps (1.3%), removal of fat necrosis (1%). Only one patient in the entire series (0.3%) required a major surgical corrective reintervention in order to remove some extensive calcified necrosis and reconstruction with bilateral implants.

Complications were primarily present in patients with obesity and a smoking habit [14].

4. Conclusions

Based on a published series of patients who intervened with this technique [14], it can be concluded that it is possible to combine the techniques of CP, autologous dermis mesh, and circumferential periareolar, all of them described in Medical Literature for reduction and/or breast pexias. The combined technique here utilized is versatile in the management of the breasts' volume and symmetry, also for mobilizing the NAC and stabilizing it with dermis mesh anchored to the pectoralis major fascia and the chest wall fascia. Also, it produces a stable, well-projected central cone, which, by being covered with skin (double layer), can achieve a breast with greater firmness.

The accumulation of periareolar skin with "Raund Block", allows to reduce the submammary scar, in order to not exceed the breast limits.

In our experience, it is a safe procedure, with few complications [14]. Because of the good irrigation and sensitivity of the CP, we can reduce major breast volumes and preserve lactation, since all the mammarian tissues of the CP are connected to the NAC. The obtained breast shape is stable in time, with minimal ptosis of the NAC and the inferior pole, achieving high satisfaction with the patients [14].

Conflict of interests

The authors declare having no financial interest related to the contents of this article. Neither have they received help or payments for the realization of this study.

Author details

Armin Rudolph Geisse[1*], Klaus Rudolph Oppliger[2] and Thomas Rudolph Oppliger[3]

1 Faculty of Medicine in Universidad de la Frontera, Temuco, Chile

2 Hospital de Toltén, Chile

3 Universidad Mayor, Temuco, Chile

*Address all correspondence to: armin.rudolph@ufrontera.cl

References

[1] Pitanguy I. Surgical treatment of breast hypertrophy. British Journal of Plastic Surgery. 1967;**20**(1):78-85

[2] Georgiade N. Reduction mammaplasty utilizing the inferior pedicle nipple-areolar flap. Annals of Plastic Surgery. 1979;**3**(3):211-212

[3] McKissock P. Reduction mammaplasty by the vertical bipedicle flap technique: Rationale and results. Clinicals of Plastic Surgery. 1976;**3**(2):309-320

[4] Balch C. The central mound technique for reduction mammaplasty. Plastic Reconstruction Surgery. 1981;**67**(3):305-311

[5] Hester T et al. Breast reduction utilizing the maximally vascularized central breast pedicle. Plastic Reconstruction Surgery. 1985;**76**(6):890-900

[6] Calderon W et al. Mamoplastía de Reducción con incisión periareolar: anatomía y clínica del pedículo central. Cir. Plást. Iberolatinoam. 2016;**42**(1):21-28

[7] White D et al. Clinical applications of the central pedicle technique of the breast reduction. Operative Techniques in Plastic and Reconstructive Surgery. 1996;**3**(3):176-183

[8] Grant J et al. The maximally vascularized central pedicle breast reduction: Evolution of a technique. Annals of Plastic Surgery. 2001;**46**:584-589

[9] See M-H. Central pedicle reduction mammaplasty: A reliable technique. Gland Surgery. 2014;**3**(1):51-54

[10] Delong M et al. The Central Mound Pedicle: A safe and effective technique for reduction mammaplasty. Plastic Reconstruction Surgery. 2020;**146**(4):725-733

[11] Góes JC. Periareolar mammaplasty: Doble skin technique with application of Polyglactine or mixed mesh. Plastic and Reconstructive Surgery. 1996;**97**(5):959-968

[12] Góes JC. Periareolar mastopexy: Doble skin technique with mesh support. Surgical Journal. 2003;**23**:129-135

[13] Benelli L. A new periareolar mammaplasty: The "Round Block" technique. Surgical Journal. 1990;**14**(2):93-100

[14] Rudolph A. Mamoplastía de reducción con Pedículo Central y Malla de Dermis. Cir. Plást. Iberolatinoam. 2021;**47**(1):35-48

[15] Yépez I. Mamoplastía de reducción con cicatrices pequeñas para grandes hipertrofias mamarias o gigantomastias. Cir. Plást. Iberolatinoam. 2013;**39**(1):1-8

[16] Souto G. The impact of breast reduction surgery on breastfeeding performance. Journal of Human Lactation. 2003;**19**(1):43-49

[17] Wirthmann A et al. Reduction mammaplasty in adolescents and elderly: A ten year case series analyzing age related outcome with focus on safety and complications. Journal of Plastic, Reconstructive & Esthetic Surgery. 2018;**71**(3):377-383

[18] Gulcelik M et al. Early complications of a reduction mammaplasty technique in the treatment of macromastia with or without breast cancer. Clinical Breast Cancer. 2011;**11**(6):395-399

[19] Fischer J et al. Complications following reduction mammaplasty: A review of 3538 cases from the 2005-2010 NSQIP data sets. Esthetic Surgery Journal. 2014;**34**(1):66-73

[20] Srinivasaiah N et al. Risk factors for complications following breast reduction: Results from a randomized control trial. The Breast Journal. 2014;**20**(3):274-278

[21] Zhang M et al. Risk factors for complications after reduction mammaplasty: A meta-analysis. PLoS One. 2016;**11**(12):e0167746

Section 4

Safety

Chapter 6

Perspective Chapter: Identification of Body Contouring Surgery Complications by Multispectral RGB/Infrared Thermography Imaging

Marcos Leal Brioschi, Soane Couto Menezes Lemos, Carlos Dalmaso Neto, Franciele De Meneck, Patricia Rodrigues Resende and Eduardo Borba Neves

Abstract

Infrared thermography can assist in the documentation of inflammatory vascular healing reactions and tissue perfusion resulting from esthetic surgical procedures in different parts of the body and face. Both in preoperative planning and in its postoperative evolutionary behavior. Infrared thermography is a functional imaging technique of cutaneous vascular activity using long-infrared electromagnetic radiation emitted by tissue cells. It can accurately identify terminal cutaneous perforating vessels related to greater or lesser skin perfusion, non-invasively, quickly, painlessly, safely and without emission of ionizing radiation by scanning a segment or entire body in a single image. This facilitates the evaluation of patients undergoing lipoabdominoplasty and their postoperative follow-up. Monitoring of new techniques and traditional procedures with infrared scanning technology helps in the early diagnostic elucidation of complications (edema, seromas, epidermolysis, hematoma, dehiscence, infection, necrosis), evolutionary studies of healing and local effects of thermoguided procedures (such as manual therapy, laser photobiomodulation, ultrasound, radiofrequency, hyperbaric oxygen therapy) direct the treatment with more objectivity, better results, and safety.

Keywords: thermography, healing, abdominoplasty, postoperative complications, abdominal wall

1. Introduction

Physiologic risks of plastic surgical procedures are comparably less than those of other surgical subspecialties, as the procedures are typically elective, and usually performed in relatively healthy subjects. Most common postoperative complications include infections, local anesthetic systemic toxicity, electrolyte and hematologic

 IntechOpen

abnormalities, intravascular fluid shifts, deep vein thrombosis, and wound complications (hematoma, ecchymosis, swelling, seroma, tissue edema, localized pain, nerve damage, infections, and cellulitis). In a lipoabdominoplasty systematic review 5.6% of wound infection, dehiscence, or fat necrosis; 4.1% of seroma; 0.8% hematoma; 0.2% deep venous thrombosis; and 0.7% scar deformity [1]. Studies on the use of thermography in the plastic surgery field are promising. Most of them verified the use of infrared thermography to assess perforating vessels' location and quality in the pre, intra- and postoperative period and concluded that the thermographic examination helps in planning the surgeries and more efficient results with a reduction in complications [2, 3].

So, it is important to review the literature regarding the use of infrared thermography, exposing how it works as a complementary functional bedside exam; and discussing what is known about the applicability of this method in abdominoplasty post-operatory complications.

2. Methods

2.1 Infrared imaging (thermography)

Infrared thermography is a non-invasive, non-contact, non-ionizing, functional imaging method for direct measurement of skin temperature surface and indirect measurement of skin perfusion, microcirculation, inflammation, metabolism, and sympathetic vasomotor nerve activity, providing a surface temperature distribution map. The assessment of skin perfusion through the identification of arterial-perforating vessels, with their location visible on thermography as skin "hot spots" [4] by thermography has been used in plastic surgery with good success. However, skin temperature and skin blood flow were not linearly correlated. While skin temperature can be used to study thermal physiology, it should not be considered a substitute for dermal blood flow.

The human body emits thermal radiation, and there is a correlation between the energy of the thermal radiation and the temperature of the skin. Infrared thermography is a method of remote scanning of the human body that identifies areas of greater or lesser brightness of infrared thermal radiation. According to the Stefan-Boltzmann law, the greater the radiation emitted by a body, the greater its temperature – $W = \varepsilon\sigma T^4$, where W is the rate of emission of infrared radiant energy (W/m^2), ε is the emissivity of the body (0.98 for the human body), σ is the Stefan-Boltzmann constant (5.7×10^{-8}Wm^{-2} K^{-4}), and T the body temperature (K). To maintain its internal thermal homeostasis, the body exchanges heat with the environment (conduction, convection, evaporation). The energy emitted in the form of infrared radiation represents 60% of the total, with 80–90% doing so with a long wavelength of 8–15 μm when the person is exposed in a room at 23°C for 15 min. The thermal transducer can detect the infrared radiation emitted by the skin surface and generate an entire body surface thermal map image.

Skin temperature depends on the cutaneous and subcutaneous tissues' vascular supply and skin thermal conductivity as it is affected in different cutaneous pathological situations. Localized blood flow changes related to capillary system alterations can induce changes in skin temperature and therefore reveal skin inflammation, ischemic areas, or cellulite [5]. Consequently, monitoring skin temperature would provide information related to the blood flow throw the skin [6].

2.2 The perforating vessels thermal concept

The subcutaneous tissue contains small and medium-sized arteries, crossing the hypodermis in two ways: a) perpendicular, where the path crosses the fascial and subcutaneous layers to reach the skin (perforating arteries); b) longitudinal, the course where they cross the subcutaneous tissue in an oblique course following the superficial fascia for extensive lengths. Vessels follow, in subcutaneous layers, the retinacula – that provides protection to vessels and prevents their displacement when the skin is pulled –, to go perpendicularly from the deepest skin planes. Around the retinacula, the vessels have a tortuous path with many curves. So, when the skin is lifted, the vessels can stretch without damage.

The areas of greatest thermal leakage correspond to the exit sites of subcutaneous axial vessels called perforating vessels, that perfuse a certain cutaneous area (angiotome). 97% of the perforating cutaneous vessels observed on Doppler ultrasound coincide with thermal points presence (hot spots on thermography) [7]. Doppler ultrasound locates perforators at a deeper level, whereas thermography locates them more superficially (under the skin surface). As such, they showed that no cold challenge may be necessary. Blood vessel expansion, and consequent flow volume increase of these perforating vessels, are sympathetic neurovegetative nervous system controlled. So, poorly myelinated sympathetic fibers control the cutaneous perfusion of their corresponding dermatome/angiossome. Cutaneous microcirculation has a thermoregulatory function, being essential for steady body temperature maintenance. Although the volume of the capillaries is small, their surface area is large compared with other skin vessels.

Physiological regulation of cutaneous microcirculation includes sympathetic activation, which causes vasoconstriction. The sympathetic cholinergic system is mainly involved in vasodilation. Endothelium-dependent vasomotion implicates nitric oxide, prostacyclin, endothelium-dependent hyperpolarizing factors, and endothelin. Variations in skin blood flow result from highly complex interactions between these mechanisms, and perfusion assessment for the impaired cutaneous blood flow early detection may alert clinicians to microvascular changes as a marker of tissue viability. In certain situations, thermal stress can be performed to produce skin cooling and vasoconstriction and, subsequently, thermal images can be obtained during the cutaneous rewarming process using the perforating cutaneous vessels [2–4, 8]. Thermography reinforces the importance of performing local healing treatment at thermal points, rather than at an arbitrary location on the skin.

The manual or bioelectrical mechanical thermal point stimulation in a richly vascularized and innervated area explains much of the local and segmental effects of post-operative care procedures, by vascular activation, and by the peripheral sensory and sympathetic neurovegetative nervous system [9]. Infrared thermography permits evolutionary studies of healing and local effects of thermoguided procedures (manual therapy, laser photobiomodulation, ultrasound, radiofrequency, hyperbaric oxygen therapy [10–12]) near perforator vessels directing treatment with more objectivity, better results, and safety.

2.3 Bedside post-surgical thermography method

Patients must be instructed to not have a hot bath less than 2 h before assessment, not to use any topical substance on the skin, fastening for at least 3 h before the exam, and not to take stimulant substances (coffee, alcohol, cigarettes, etc.) 10 h before examination. An infrared thermography exam is usually performed 24 to 48 h postoperatively, before hospital discharge, and on the 5th, 25th, and 27th day after the operation. Captured thermal images are obtained using a double spectroscopy infrared-visual camera, 320x240 pixels image resolution, thermal sensitivity of 0.05°C and cutaneous emissivity set at 0.98, in a room with 23 ± 1°C controlled temperature, relative humidity less than 60%, and minimum air convection of 0.2 m/s. Patients rest comfortably, without abdomen covering clothes. First images should be taken 15 min after dressing removal, and captured at approximately 50 cm at straight angles. These images, in the double spectroscopy mode, are processed using specific color scales and oriented to a three-dimensional qualitative study using the Hypermax® function (**Figure 1C**, **F**, **I** and **L**; **Figure 2C**; **Figure 3C** and **F**; **Figure 4** and **Figure 5C**, **F** and **I**),

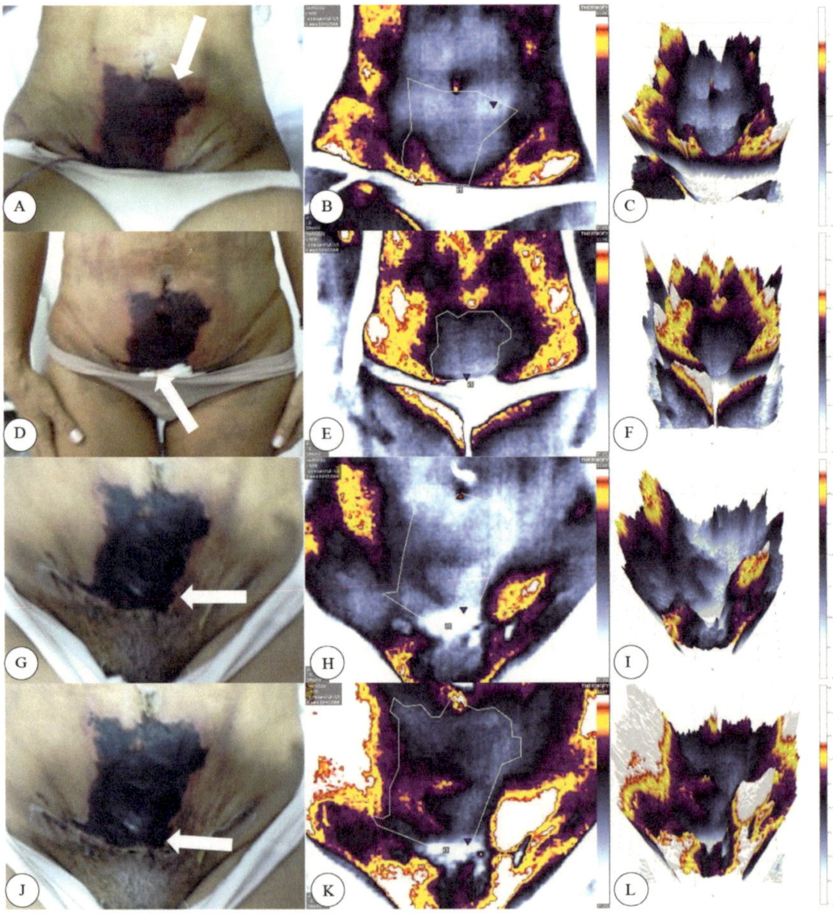

Figure 1.
Patient undergoing liposuction associated with mini-abdominoplasty and diastasis correction. On the 2nd POD progressed to infraumbilical pain and burning sensation, and the strap was removed. An area of possible tissue suffering was observed (B-C). Immediate indications for hyperbaric and ozone therapy to delimit the area and surrounding tissue oxygenation. Thermographic follow-up on subsequent days maintenance of daily hyperbaric therapy and ozone therapy on alternate days (via bag) in the abdominal region. On the 7th POD, showing delimited epidermolysis and central necrosis (D-F). On 12th POD, a change in the tissue appearance (G) (carapace more rigid in the lower third) evolving with dehiscence in the scar area, with correspondent hyporadiation (H-I). Initial option of autolytic debridement and special dressings (vacuum) to prepare for future corrective surgical intervention. Hyporadiation area (K-L) smaller than before (B).

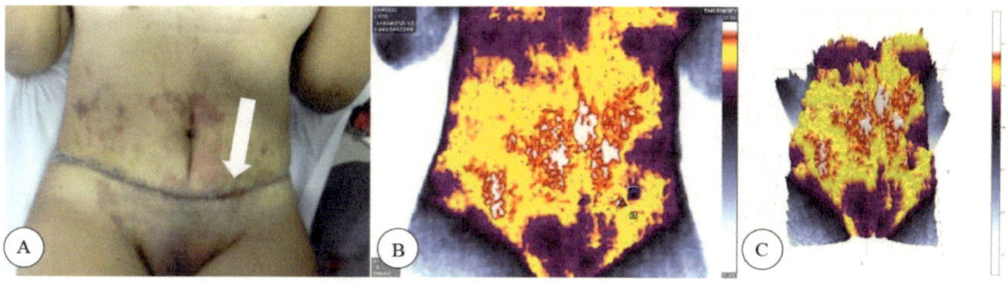

Figure 2.
Another patient undergoing lipoabdominoplasty, with diastasis correction on the 5th POD, with ecchymosis areas (burn, hemosiderin deposition), without signs of pain or local burning. Thermographic imaging (A) helped in the conservative management choice in the abdomen, and therapy in a small hyporadiant cold area at the scar (left iliac fossa) (B). After removal of the surgical glue, the patient presented with an intact scar, and the skin evolved only with brownish spots.

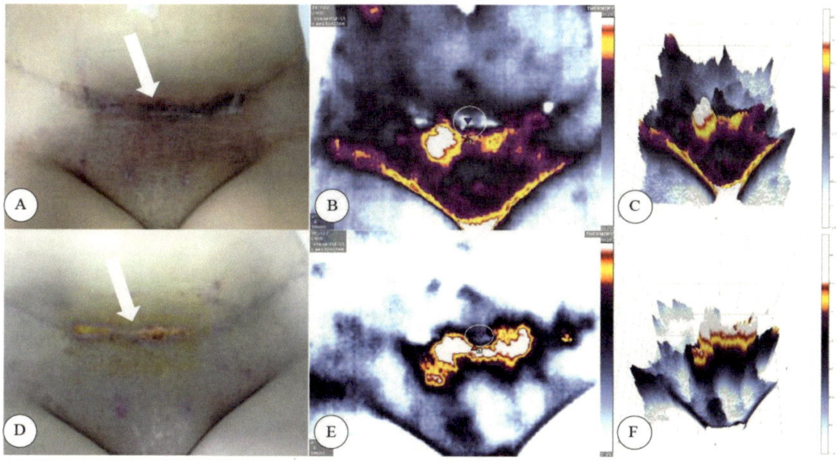

Figure 3.
Patient on the 8th POD of reduction mammoplasty and abdominoplasty scar correction performed 1 month early. When using surgical glue, it is possible to identify cold-hyporadiating areas (A, B, and C), with possible dehiscence. Tissue repair therapy with photobiomodulation, manual therapy, and local ozone therapy was started (D, E and F), 2 days after the first images.

and quantitative study using automated tables and graphs of authors developed specific software (VisionFy®, Thermofy, Brazil).

With the development and greater precision of infrared transducers, it is now possible to combine them with automatic evaluation through medical analysis software and obtain automatic recording in real-time, with high precision, establishing the continuous dynamics of certain thermal points, and the immediate and late effect of local post-surgical healing treatment.

The image analysis process extracts parameters describing the overall skin temperature (median T°; T° amplitude), the homogeneity of the temperature (Sa, Sz, Sq), and the visual contrast between hot and cold areas on the images (number and surface of cold and hot areas). Standard roughness parameters (Ra, Rz, Rq) are extracted from these images to capture the changes in skin temperature homogeneity – Roughness Average (Ra) is the arithmetic average of the absolute profile heights T values over the evaluation length; Average Maximum Height of the Profile (Rz) is the T average of the successive values of RT_i calculated over the evaluation length.

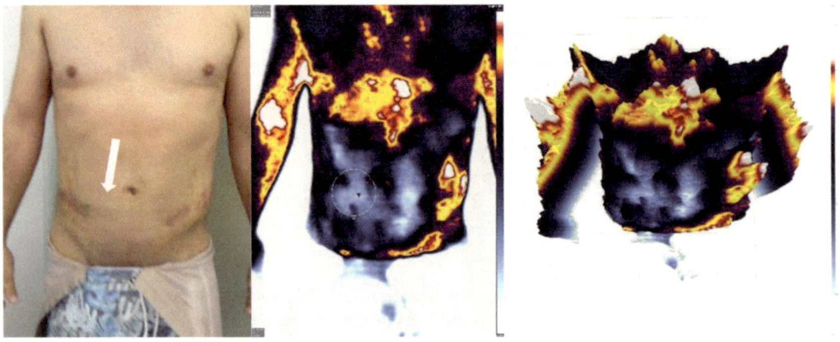

Figure 4.
Patient in the first week of high-definition liposuction, presented with hyporadiant area in the right flank and iliac fossa, with seroma-suggestive signs. No pain or other inflammatory signs.

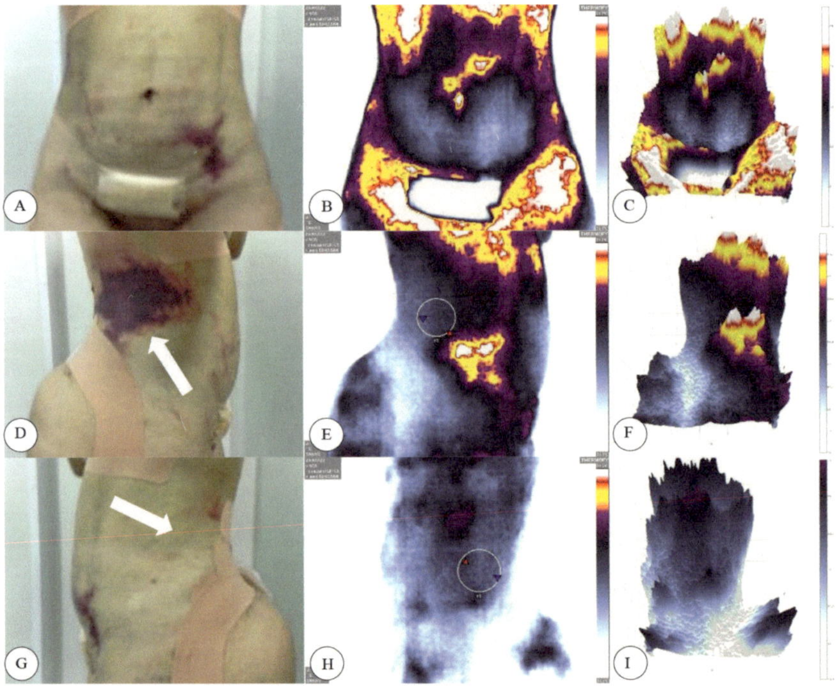

Figure 5.
Patient on the 5th POD of definition liposuction, using a device to promote skin retraction. Started hyperbaric therapy on the 1st POD. A-C, showing the frontal view, D-F right view, and G-I left view. The iliac fossa area evolved only with hypercromia, without necrosis and tissue loss. Area of intense ecchymosis (showed in D), evolved later to an area already identified with necrosis (past 11th POD). The left area evolved only with hyperchromia, with no signs of necrosis and tissue loss.

RMS Roughness (Rq) is the profile height T root mean square average over the evaluation length. The scale proposed in the literature evolves from a uniform hot skin to a "leopard" pattern skin and finally to a uniform cold skin. Thus, the overall skin temperature and homogeneity are related to skin complications.

For thermal image analysis, in the case of lipoabdominoplasy, Huger zones, reviewed by Matarasso [13], can be used as a region of interest (ROI) reference, which considers the anterior abdominal wall vascular anatomy and that region's blood supply.

The ROI SA3 (caution) was chosen, where two ROIs were determined in this area: ROI_1, at the highest point (supra umbilical); and ROI_2, at the lowest point above the suture, due to random and axial blood supply to the abdomen. To assess complications risk due to ischemia or tissue inflammation the values of the delta-R (ΔT_R), and difference in minimum ROI_1 temperature with minimum ROI_2 temperature were calculated.

3. Results

3.1 Hyperradiant areas (inflammation, infection)

Resende et al. [14] published the results of two clinical cases with thermal imaging monitoring of lipoabdominoplasty healing process, in the immediate postoperative evaluation, using the delta-R methodology: 1) ΔT_R = 0.4°C on 1st postoperative date (POD), decreasing to 0.1°C on 5th POD, without complications; and 2) ΔT_R = 1.7°C on 1st POD, remained high (ΔT_R = 2.2°C) on 5th POD (evolving to surgical scar necrosis). ΔT_R thermal index may be a new tool for predicting possible complications, complementing the clinical evaluation, and therapeutic decision-making was the conclusion.

Cicatricial complications in Plastic Surgery can arise from blood stagnation (thermographically represented by greater energy leakage), which can be generated by a local, systemic etiological factor, or a combination of these. In tissue ischemia, there is a decrease in tissue perfusion and local oxygen diffusion, causing a deficiency of elements responsible for cellular mitochondrial metabolism, and the typical sensation of discomfort, heaviness, or pain. This blockage can be aggravated by bad positioned external compressive factors presence (compression mesh and abdominal splints) or local infectious factors that prolong and accentuate the process. More than 90% of O_2 consumption in humans is due to mitochondrial metabolism, which is used to generate ATP, which fuels cellular processes such as during wound healing, and generates tissue repair energy, which consequently leads to a hypermetabolic state. About 55% of the energy is lost as heat, the rest in enzymatic-cell reactions. Every time the chemical energy contained in ATP molecules is transferred to the functional systems of cells, more energy is dissipated as heat. Also, ATP induces endothelium-dependent vasodilation. Acute inflammation following the injury process (NADPH oxidases and nitric-oxide synthases related) also produces more heat. Therefore, skin temperature increase in the initial healing process is normal and expected.

Therapeutic post-surgical techniques consist of manual and physical means of application on the body surface, to restore tissue healing, energy balance of this system, and promote remission of post-operative symptoms, and thermography has been used in the therapeutic application of plastic surgery, diagnosis, and selection of cutaneous perforating vascular points to being closely stimulated, as well as for real-time assessment of the immediate effects produced by patient's rehabilitation intervention and reassessment. There is a temperature gradient between the thermal spot location and the surrounding tissue, that is, there is a significant thermal difference between the location of the spot and the neighboring tissue [15].

3.2 Hyporadiant areas (swelling, seroma, epidermolysis, hematoma, necrosis, dehiscence, fibrosis)

Normal abdominal surface infrared emission usually has a mottled pattern of heat gradations, normally varying about 1°C. In the central region, there is a hot spot caused by the depression imprinted by the umbilicus cross-radiation. The underlying areas of fat are good insulators and tend to decrease skin temperature as they become thicker. Places of blood accumulation, such as bruises or very inflamed skin, raise the skin temperature locally. In contrast, benign processes, and other regions of low metabolic activity, such as hair, seromas, epidermolysis, ecchymosis, gangrene, dehiscence, and necrotic tissue, are hyporadiant (**Figure 1B**, **E**, **H**, and **K**; **Figure 2B** and **E**).

Temperature differences between wound and reference skin territories could provide a possible infection risk thermal "signature", with "cold spots" proposed as a marker of an "avascular" region along the incision site [16]. The maximum temperature difference between healthy reference abdominal skin and wound site exceeds 2°C in developing surgical site infection (SSI) suspects. 1°C reduction in abdominal temperature led to a 3-fold raised odds of infection. A 1°C temperature widening between ROI_2–ROI_1 (wound minus abdomen) was associated with an odds ratio for SSI of 2.25 (on day 2) and 2.5 (on day 7) [17]. "Cold spots", due to a reduction in cutaneous blood flow, were observed along the scar from day 2 in many women who later developed SSI (wound being observed "hotter" than the abdomen on the thermal image).

Cutaneous necrosis in abdominoplasty can be presented visually simply, as signs of self-limited epidermolysis and small dehiscence until extensive necrosis with loss of substances in deep planes [13]. In the immediate postoperative period, the expected physiological effect is an increase in blood flow, with a consequent increase in temperature, the inflammatory process inherent to tissue healing. The normally expected drop in the wound infrared emission occurs 1 to 3 days before the rapid increase in tensile strength. Temperature peak coincides with the increase in mucopolysaccharides in the scar (**Figure 3A** and **D**), an essential component for collagen formation. A decrease in infrared emission is associated with the "collagen phase" of wound healing. In the case of infection or wound dehiscence, there is a prolongation or plateau of infrared emission, indicating a delay in healing.

It is possible to use thermal imaging to detect accentuated hyporadiation, as observed in **Figure 3** and, consequently, a situation of decreased perfusion is much more sensitive than visual or tactile clinical evaluation. Only the central area progressed to superficial necrosis, which justified maintenance of conservative care (bandages) without surgical intervention (different from **Figure 1** case). There is always the possibility of reducing blood flow in the region surrounding the surgical incision, with consequent impairment of oxygenation and nutrients delivery to the wound, so the authors suggest calculating the delta-R (ΔT_R) in SA3 region using the minimum temperature between ROIs 1 and 2, as between these areas the main angiosomes and perforating vessels responsible for the nutrition of the flap (critical area) are located [13]. In any surgery, there is a possibility of reducing blood flow in the specific region to the surgical incision, with consequent impairment in oxygenation and delivery of nutrients to the wound. The importance of checking reference values for normal and pathological deltas (such as ΔT_R) in early monitoring of the healing process in plastic surgery is emphasized to serve as safer parameters for early decision-making.

Subcutaneous fat may be related to postoperative wound complications. Abdominal subcutaneous tissue thickness represents a significant risk factor for infection in the abdominal wound incision region [18]. Using the gold standard Dual-Energy X-Ray Absorptiometry (DXA) and bioelectrical impedance with infrared thermography [19, 20], women exhibit lower values of surface temperature than males on the abdomen, which was related to a higher body fat percentage in this gender. Higher body fat percentages are related to lower skin surface temperature in the abdomen. It appears to be a greater risk of infectious complications in the cooler abdominal wall, in women.

The adipose tissue affects heat emission processes in obese women because the skin microcirculation is impaired in these areas (vessels <150 μm in diameter). Larger fat lobes decrease local vascularity. In the large-deposit white adipose tissue, essentially peri-umbilical, cells are concentrated and linked by a weak net of collagen fibers. Collagenic components are very poor, cells are large (95 μm) and few blood vessels are present. There is a structural absence of capillaries and arterioles, and the microcirculation is formed by thin-walled capillaries with rare stem niches [21]. The subcutaneous region also includes the venous plexus which strongly influences skin temperature. Poorly vascularized areas of those rich in fat tissue have a lower temperature.

We observed that the seroma and hematoma presence are usually hyporadiating in thermal images (**Figure 4**), and have a more diffuse distribution, not limited to the anatomical area and the angiosomes of that region (**Figures 4** and **5**). Greater differences in temperature (ΔT_R) may suggest, in addition to the impairment of microcirculation and metabolic tissue activity, more serious complications are, and worse the prognosis. In lipoabdominoplasty postoperative period, hyporadiating areas were related to microcirculatory complications (hematomas and seromas). Greater temperature differences in the caution area may suggest necrosis. It is recommended to avoid excessive liposuction, closure under tension, and very tight compressive meshes use, to reduce the risk of ischemia [1, 22]. Similarly, edema formation and liquid stasis in the extravascular spaces should be avoided (as they can lead to the plugging of small local vessels) [23]. It is important to remark that the meshes fold in the abdomen midline, regardless of the type of compressive mesh used; these folds can exert greater pressure on the midline of the abdomen and can decrease blood flow [13].

Long arteries are usually connected by long anastomoses, which form longitudinal arches arranged in the deep subcutaneous fat tissue. All the capillaries of the fat lobules originate from these oblique arteries. Subcutaneous tissue is arranged in anatomical units or compartments, and each anatomical compartment is associated with an identifiable artery and vein [24]. These compartments could correspond to the abdominal quadrants, and the specific organization of the superficial fascia and retinaculum cutis defines the subcutaneous compartments, and the distribution of these vessels.

All subcutaneous arteries participate in the formation of two freely communicating subcutaneous plexuses: the subpapillary plexus, just below the papillary dermis; and the deep plexus, within the superficial fascia. Only one-fifth of the capillaries are needed for skin vascularization, while the others involve thermoregulation function. The deep plexus arteries have many arteriovenous connections, that provide shunts that control blood flow to the skin and, consequently, regulate body temperature. Dilation and narrowing of subcutaneous arteries determine skin temperature and color. The marked pallor of the skin seen in acute shock is a result of the vasoconstriction of the arterial plexus in the hypodermis. It can be assumed that a fibrotic superficial fascia over time could suffocate the arteries within it, thus changing skin color or even chronic skin ischemia. Chronic ischemia can increase subcutaneous fibrosis, creating a vicious circle, and persistent cutaneous cooling, with a well-defined local hyporadiation. If arteriovenous shunts become deficient, thermoregulation change may occur, thus resulting in sensations of excessively hot or cold skin.

4. Discussion

A selection of healthy thermal points for therapeutic treatment with thermographic support, compared with the conventional blind treatment, without the use of thermography in the postoperative abdominoplasty period, was examinate. The thermo-assisted group had a reduced number of sessions, complications, and shorter treatment duration in our experience. Additionally, studies have been conducted in which the diagnosis is obtained according to the symptoms and thermographic images in the patient's pain area. Based on this assessment, selected points distant from the patient's pain area were selected for the local heat treatment application, while using thermal imaging, to objectively observe the temperature modulation, with a rise between 0.5°C and 2°C in the cold symptomatic area and decrease in the inflammatory, coinciding with pain relief (**Figures 1–5**).

Recently, other non-invasive means have shown promise for treating postoperative complications as they do not cause pain and increase local microcirculation with increased temperature when applied to thermal points. Thermal imaging ROI showed that additional stimulation with a multimodal infrared light-emitting diode (IR-LED) pad (700 nm to 1000 nm range) caused 113% increase in temperature, compared to stimulation without IR-LED. Photobiomodulation had significant effects on cutaneous vascular stimulation.

Infrared thermography can be the key to identifying specifically the main limitations of a given wound, by evaluating its vascular tone. For example, the supply of oxygen and nutrients to the wound bed is provided by adequate blood flow to the healing site, whereas hypoxia delays healing. Reduced blood flow in the surrounding wound incision region causes a disbalance in oxygen and nutrients delivery to the wound, adding slow wound healing risk, or infection, by creating areas of skin commensurate with "low-perfusion". Wound pO_2 correction alone can trigger healing responses such as vascular endothelial growth factor expression, angiogenesis, and fibroblast stimulation, as optimizing wound perfusion provides supplemental O_2 that reduces the incidence of postoperative infections [25].

Chronic ischemic wounds are essentially hypoxic, which is incompatible with tissue repair. Among the causes that can decrease the temperature at the lipoabdominoplasty site, and cause moderate-to-mild hypoxia, is a sympathetic response to pain, hypothermia, and anemia, caused by major blood loss. Tissue at the near-anoxic sites will be vulnerable to necrosis, that in turn may propagate secondary tissue damage and infection. These areas of low perfusion and oxygenation, vascular "dead-space" region, possibly due to seroma or edema, may be heterogeneously distributed in the surgical site, creating true pockets with different levels of hypoxia. It is important to identify these cold spots through thermography as irregular cold "islands" distributed throughout the abdomen; and to thermally compare these areas with normal areas, as located within a higher average temperature, and blood flow, wound region, by averaging the temperature values.

Analyzing the extent and number of "islands" of low temperature within the wound, with the contribution of the adjacent healthy abdominal temperature, will improve the early identification of tissue complications. By mapping the abdominal wall skin temperature using thermal imaging, the aim is to assess the subtle changes in wound skin perfusion/oxygenation, and adjacent tissues, in the first days after surgery. The objective is to anticipate the signs and symptoms regarding post-surgical complications of infectious or non-infectious origin. There is still a lot to study about how to prevent post-plastic surgery complications. Measuring skin temperature by thermography to assess wound blood flow, and adjacent thermal territories, has the potential, as a non-invasive, independent imaging option, to identify "at risk" tissue. "Hot" or "cold" skin spot identification, proportional to regions of high or low blood flow/hypoxia, has the potential to shed light on the underlying mechanisms that lead to infectious and non-infectious wound complications.

The knowledge of the relationship between emitted long-wave thermal radiation, skin temperature, and blood flow in the abdominal incision region can offer a practical bedside functional imaging solution to broaden assessment criteria for wound prognosis from the visible spectrum to the infrared region.

Observing the wound map in "infrared", and measuring the temperature of the abdominal territories, offers a new perspective on wound assessment with an easy-to-perform technique as a complementary propaedeutic approach to exploring cutaneous microcirculation/hypoxia. Therefore, the authors of this study believe that surgeons and researchers consider the use of infrared thermography in post-operative abdominoplasty, to study the healing tissue and, if thermally identified, perform early intervention to avoid major complications.

Conflict of interests

All authors declare that they have no conflicts of interest.

Author details

Marcos Leal Brioschi[1*], Soane Couto Menezes Lemos[2], Carlos Dalmaso Neto[1,3], Franciele De Meneck[4], Patricia Rodrigues Resende[1] and Eduardo Borba Neves[5]

1 Graduate Program in Thermology and Medical Thermography, Hospital das Clínicas, Faculty of Medicine, University of São Paulo, São Paulo, Brazil

2 Physiotherapy Department, Brazilian Medical Thermology Association, Anhanguera College, Salvador, Brazil

3 Mechanical Engineering Department, Brazilian Medical Thermology Association, Federal University of Parana, Curitiba, Brazil

4 Medical Science, Federal University of Sao Paulo, São Paulo, Brazil

5 Graduate Program in Biomedical Engineering, Federal Technological University of Paraná, Curitiba, Brazil

*Address all correspondence to: termometria@yahoo.com.br

References

[1] Xia Y, Zhao J, Cao DS. Safety of Lipoabdominoplasty versus abdominoplasty: A systematic review and meta-analysis. Aesthetic Plastic Surgery. 2019;**43**(1):167-174. DOI: 10.1007/s00266-018-1270-3

[2] Cifuentes IJ, Dagnino BL, Salisbury MC, Perez ME, Ortega C, Maldonado D. Augmented reality and dynamic infrared thermography for perforator mapping in the anterolateral thigh. Archives of Plastic Surgery. 2018;**45**(03):284-288. DOI: 10.5999/aps.2017.01375

[3] Hennessy O, Potter SM. Use of infrared thermography for the assessment of free flap perforators in autologous breast reconstruction: A systematic review. JPRAS Open. 2020;**23**:60-70. DOI: 10.1016/j.jpra.2019.11.006

[4] de Weerd L, Miland ÅO, Mercer JB. Perfusion dynamics of free DIEP and SIEA flaps during the first postoperative week monitored with dynamic infrared thermography. Annals of Plastic Surgery. 2009;**62**(1):42-47. DOI: 10.1097/SAP.0b013e3181776374

[5] Nkengne A, Papillon A, Bertin C. Evaluation of the cellulite using a thermal infra-red camera. Skin Research and Technology. 2013;**19**(1):e231-e237. DOI: 10.1111/j.1600-0846.2012.00633.x

[6] Ammer K, Ring EFJ. Standard procedures for infrared imaging in medicine. In: Diakides M, Bronzino JD, Peterson DR, editors. organizadores. Medical Infrared Imaging. Boca Raton, FL: CRC Press; 2008. pp. 32.1-32.14

[7] Sheena Y, Jennison T, Hardwicke JT, Titley OG. Detection of perforators using thermal imaging. Plastic and Reconstructive Surgery. 2013;**132**(6):1603-1610. DOI: 10.1097/PRS.0b013e3182a80740

[8] Chubb DP, Taylor GI, Ashton MW. True and "choke" anastomoses between perforator Angiosomes: Part II. Dynamic thermographic identification. Plastic and Reconstructive Surgery. 2013;**132**(6):1457-1464. DOI: 10.1097/01.prs.0000434407.73390.82

[9] Lund I, Lundeberg T. Effects triggered in the periphery by acupuncture. Acupuncture and Related Therapies. 2015;**3**(2-3):24-34. DOI: 10.1016/j.arthe.2015.08.002

[10] Fidut-Wrońska J, Chołuj K, Chmiel J, Pikto-Pitkiewicz K, Majcher P. Observation using thermography of post-operative reaction after fascial manipulation®. Annals of Agricultural and Environmental Medicine. 2019;**26**(3):468-471. DOI: 10.26444/aaem/103456

[11] de Oliveira ME, Da Silva JT, Brioschi ML, Chacur M. Effects of photobiomodulation therapy on neuropathic pain in rats: Evaluation of nociceptive mediators and infrared thermography. Lasers in Medical Science. 2021;**36**(7):1461-1467. DOI: 10.1007/s10103-020-03187-9

[12] Key DJ. Preliminary demonstration using localized skin temperature elevation as observed with thermal imaging as an indicator of fat-specific absorption during focused-field radiofrequency therapy. Journal of Drugs Dermatology. 2014;**13**(7):864-866. DOI: 25007372

[13] Matarasso A. Classification and patient selection in abdominoplasty.

Operative Techniques in Plastic and Reconstructive Surgery. 1996;**3**(1):7-14. DOI: 10.1016/S1071-0949(96)80044-8

[14] Resende PR, Brioschi ML, De Meneck F, Neves EB, Teixeira MJ, Meneck F De, et al. Predicting lipoabdominoplasty complications with infrared thermography: A delta-R analysis. Archives of Plastic Surgery 19 de setembro de 2021;48(05):553-558. DOI: 10.5999/aps.2021.00101

[15] Wu ZYY, Liu XLL, Hong WXX, Zhang D. Research on the correlation between the temperature asymmetry at acupoints of healthy and affected side and the severity index of facial paralysis. Zhongguo Zhen Jiu. 2010;**30**(11):953-956. DOI: 21246857

[16] Childs C, Siraj MR, Fair FJ, Selvan AN, Soltani H, Wilmott J, et al. Thermal territories of the abdomen after caesarean section birth: Infrared thermography and analysis. Journal of Wound Care. 2016;**25**(9):499-512. DOI: 10.12968/jowc.2016.25.9.499

[17] Childs C, Wright N, Willmott J, Davies M, Kilner K, Ousey K, et al. The surgical wound in infrared: Thermographic profiles and early stage test-accuracy to predict surgical site infection in obese women during the first 30 days after caesarean section. Antimicrobial Resistance and Infection Control. 2019;**8**(1):1-16. DOI: 10.1186/s13756-018-0461-7

[18] Soper DE, Bump RC, Hurt WG. Wound infection after abdominal hysterectomy: Effect of the depth of subcutaneous tissue. American Journal of Obstetrics and Gynecology. 1995;**173**(2):465-471. DOI: 10.1016/0002-9378(95)90267-8

[19] Neves EB, Brioschi ML. Is it possible to use low-cost infrared cameras (thermal resolution of 80x60 pixels) in medical applications? Pan American Journal of Medical Thermology. 2017;**1**:5-6

[20] Chudecka M, Lubkowska A, Leźnicka K, Krupecki K. The use of thermal imaging in the evaluation of the symmetry of muscle activity in various types of exercises (symmetrical and asymmetrical). Journal of Human Kinetics. 2015;**49**(1):141-147. DOI: 10.1515/hukin-2015-0116

[21] Sbarbati A, Accorsi D, Benati D, Marchetti L, Orsini G, Rigotti G, et al. Subcutaneous adipose tissue classification. European Journal of Histochemistry. 2010;**54**(4):48. DOI: 10.4081/ejh.2010.e48

[22] Ardehali B, Fiorentino F. A meta-analysis of the effects of abdominoplasty modifications on the incidence of postoperative seroma. Aesthetic Surgery Journal. 2017;**37**(10):1136-1143. DOI: 10.1093/asj/sjx051

[23] Rangaswamy M. Minimising complications in abdominoplasty: An approach based on the root cause analysis and focused preventive steps. Indian Journal of Plastic Surgery. 2013;**46**(2):365. DOI: 10.4103/0970-0358.118615

[24] Schaverien MV, Coroneos CJ. Surgical treatment of lymphedema. Plastic and Reconstructive Surgery. 2019;**144**(3):738-758. DOI: 10.1097/PRS.0000000000005993

[25] Kurz A, Sessler DI, Lenhardt R. Perioperative Normothermia to reduce the incidence of surgical-wound infection and shorten hospitalization. The New England Journal of Medicine. 1996;**334**(19):1209-1216. DOI: 10.1056/NEJM199605093341901